NCLEX-RN®
MEDICATIONS
YOU NEED TO KNOW
FOR THE EXAM

RELATED KAPLAN BOOKS FOR NURSES

NCLEX-RN® Strategies, Practice, and Review
Your Career in Nursing
Medical Terms for Nurses
Math for Nurses
CCRN®

NCLEX-RN®
MEDICATIONS
YOU NEED TO KNOW
FOR THE EXAM

FOURTH EDITION

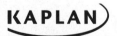

PUBLISHING

New York

Contributing Writer: Margaret A. Tiemann RN, BS

© 2011 by Kaplan, Inc.

Published by Kaplan Publishing, a division of Kaplan, Inc.
395 Hudson Street
New York, NY 10014

Printed in the United States of America

10 9 8 7 6 5 4

ISBN 13: 978-1-60714-665-0

TABLE OF CONTENTS

The following categories have been included in the book, listed in alphabetical order by category.

Allergy and Asthma Medications...........................1
Analgesics...11
Anticoagulants...23
Anticonvulsants..25
Anti-Infectives..35
Anti-Inflammatory Medications..........................71
Antineoplastics..77
Cardiovascular Medications.............................79
Dermatologicals.......................................137
Diabetic Medications..................................141
Gastrointestinal Medications..........................155
Genitourinary Medications.............................181
Hormones/Synthetic Substitutes/Modifiers..............191
Mental Health Medications.............................195
Musculoskeletal Medications...........................227
Neurological Medications..............................241
Ophthalmics...249
Respiratory Medications...............................259
Treatment/Replacement.................................271
Women's Health..285

Appendixes
JCAHO List of "Do Not Use"
   Abbreviations......................................301
Controlled Substance Schedules........................303
Pregnancy Risk Categories.............................304
Common Medical Abbreviations..........................305

HOW TO USE THIS BOOK

Kaplan NCLEX-RN® Medications You Need to Know is perfectly designed to help you learn important information about 300 essential medications in a quick, easy, and fun way. Simply read the medication's category and subcategory, generic and brand names, and the phonetic pronunciation of the generic name on the front of each page; then flip to the back to see its side effects, usage, and important nursing considerations.

Looking for still more NCLEX-RN® exam prep? Be sure to pick up a copy of Kaplan's *NCLEX-RN®: Strategies, Practice, and Review,* complete with two practice tests.

Good luck!

DISCLAIMER

The material in this book is intended for study and test-preparation purposes only. This book is under no circumstances to be used to prescribe medication, provide medical treatment and/or therapy, or treat patients or any other individuals in any way. The publisher is not responsible for use of this book in any manner other than their intended purpose as a study guide.

CETIRIZINE HCL
(se-<u>teer</u>-a-zene)

(Zyrtec)

• •

FEXOFENADINE
(fex-oh-<u>fi</u>-na-deen)

(Allegra)

Side Effects

Drowsiness	Dry mouth	Diarrhea
Fatigue	Stomach pain	Vomiting

Nursing Considerations

- Relief of seasonal allergic rhinitis symptoms
- Relief of perennial allergic rhinitis caused by molds, animal dander, and other allergens
- Avoid alcohol during cetirizine therapy
- Call physician immediately for difficulty breathing or swallowing
- Notify physician for hydroxyzine (Vistaril) allergy
- Rx; Preg Cat B

• •

Side Effects

Drowsiness	Pain	Difficulty breathing
Headache	Cough	Hoarseness
Dizziness	Hives	Swelling
Diarrhea	Rash	
Vomiting	Itching	

Nursing Considerations

- Management of rhinitis, allergy symptoms, chronic idiopathic urticaria
- Avoid alcohol, CNS depressants
- 60 mg tablet: onset within 1 hour, peak 2–3 hours, duration about 12 hours
- 180 mg tablet: duration 24 hours
- Notify physician if taking erythromycin or ketoconazole (Nizoral)
- If taking aluminum magnesium antacid, take antacid a few hours before or after fexofenadine
- Rx; Preg Cat C

HYDROXYZINE
(hye-<u>drox</u>-i-zeen)
(Anx, Atarax, Vistaril)

· ·

LORATADINE
(lor-<u>a</u>-ti-deen)
(Alavert, Claritin)

Side Effects

Drowsiness	Dizziness	Reddening of skin
Dry mouth, nose, and throat	Headache	
	Chest congestion	

Nursing Considerations

- Treatment of pruritus, pre-op anxiety, post-op nausea and vomiting, to potentiate opioid analgesics, sedation
- PO: onset 15–30 minutes, duration 4–6 hours
- Avoid use with alcohol, CNS depressants
- Teach patient that dizziness/drowsiness may occur; use caution in potentially hazardous activities
- Treatment of symptoms of alcohol withdrawal
- Notify physician of diagnosis of glaucoma, ulcers, enlarged prostate gland, liver disease, hypertension, seizures, or hyperthyroidism
- Observe for difficulty breathing
- Muscle weakness
- Increased anxiety
- Rx; Preg Cat C

• •

Side Effects

Headache	Nervousness	Hives
Dry mouth	Weakness	Swelling of face or extremities
Epistaxis (nosebleed)	Stomach pain	
Sore throat	Wheezing	Hoarseness
Diarrhea	Dysphagia	Mouth sores
Rash	Dyspnea	Insomnia

Nursing Considerations

- Management of seasonal rhinitis
- Avoid alcohol, CNS depressants
- Take on empty stomach 1 hour before or 2 hours after meals
- Onset 1–3 hours, peak 8–12 hours, duration ≥ 24 hours
- OTC, Rx; Preg Cat B

BECLOMETHASONE
(be-kloe-<u>meth</u>-a-sone)
(Beclovent, Beconase, Qvar)

• •

FLUNISOLIDE
(floo-<u>niss</u>-oh-lide)
(Aerobid, Nasalide)

Side Effects

Dysphonia	Sore throat	Nausea
Hoarseness	Dyspepsia	Cough
Oropharyngeal fungal infections	Unpleasant taste and smell	Angioedema
Headache	Rhinitis	Back pain

Nursing Considerations

- Used in chronic asthma treatment, seasonal or perennial rhinitis
- Prevention of recurrence of nasal polyps after surgical removal
- Nasal spray: onset 5–7 days (up to 3 weeks in some patients), peak up to 3 weeks
- Inhaler: onset 10 minutes
- Use regular peak flow monitoring to determine respiratory status
- Rx; Preg Cat C

• •

Side Effects

Dysphonia	Sore throat	Unpleasant taste, upset stomach
Hoarseness	Nasal congestion, cold symptoms	Epistaxis (nosebleed)
Oropharyngeal fungal infections	Nausea, vomiting, diarrhea	
Headache		

Nursing Considerations

- Used in chronic asthma treatment, seasonal or perennial rhinitis
- Onset: few days
- Use regular peak flow monitoring to determine respiratory status
- Rx; Preg Cat C

FLUTICASONE

(floo-<u>tik</u>-a-sone)

(Flonase)

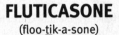

FLUTICASON PROPIONATE
SALMETROL

(floo-<u>tik</u>-a-sone <u>proe</u>-pee-oh-nate sal-<u>me</u>-te-rol)

(Advair Diskus)

Side Effects

Dysphonia

Hoarseness

Oropharyngeal fungal infections

Headache

Sore throat

Nasal congestion, cold symptoms

Nausea, vomiting, diarrhea

Unpleasant taste, upset stomach

Epistaxis (nosebleed), nasal irritation

Hives

Dyspnea

Dysphagia

Angioedema

Nursing Considerations

- Used in chronic asthma treatment, seasonal or perennial rhinitis
- Nasal spray: onset within 2 days, peak 1–2 weeks
- Use regular peak flow monitoring to determine respiratory status
- Rx; Preg Cat C

• •

Side Effects

Nausea, vomiting, diarrhea

Headache

Dysphonia, hoarseness

Throat irritation, cough

Oropharyngeal fungal infections

Muscle and bone pain

Viral respiratory infections, bronchitis

Nursing Considerations

- Used when asthma is not well controlled with long-term inhaled corticosteroids; COPD
- Oral inhalation; rinse mouth with water after inhalation
- Twice-daily dosage, 12 hours apart; used long term
- Use regular peak flow monitoring to determine respiratory status
- Monitor growth of pediatric patient
- Monitor for glaucoma and cataracts
- May decrease bone mineral density
- Monitor for eosinophilic conditions, hypokalemia, and hyperglycemia
- May increase risk of pneumonia in patients with COPD
- May cause worsening of infections
- Check oral cavity for *Candida albicans*
- Rx; Preg Cat C

MOMETASONE
(moe-<u>met</u>-a-sone)

(Nasonex Spray)

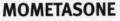

Allergy and Asthma Medications
Corticosteroids

TRIAMCINOLONE
(trye-am-<u>sin</u>-oh-lone)

(Nasacort AQ Spray)

Side Effects

Dysphonia
Hoarseness
Oropharyngeal fungal infections
Headache
Sore throat

Nasal congestion, cold
  symptoms
Nausea, vomiting, diarrhea
Unpleasant taste, upset stomach

Nursing Considerations

- Used in chronic asthma treatment, seasonal or perennial rhinitis
- Nasal spray: onset few days, peak up to 3 weeks
- Use regular peak flow monitoring to determine respiratory status
- Rx; Preg Cat C

• •

Side Effects

Dysphonia; hoarseness
Oropharyngeal fungal infections
Headache
Sore throat
Nasal congestion, cold
  symptoms

Nausea, vomiting, diarrhea
Unpleasant taste, upset stomach
Epistaxis (nosebleed)
Flu syndrome
Increased cough
Bronchitis

Nursing Considerations

- Used in chronic asthma treatment, seasonal or perennial rhinitis
- Nasal spray: onset few days, peak 3–4 days
- PO/IM: peak 1–2 hours
- Use regular peak flow monitoring to determine respiratory status
- Rx; Preg Cat C

ACETAMINOPHEN
(a-seat-a-<u>mee</u>-noe-fen)

(Acephen, Enducet, FeverAll, Genapap, Genebs, Liquiprin, Tylenol, Wygesic)

• •

ASPIRIN
(<u>as</u>-pir-in)

Side Effects

Anemia (long-term use) Angioedema
Liver and kidney failure Hives, itching
Dyspnea (high prolonged doses)

Nursing Considerations

- Treatment of mild pain or fever
- PO: onset less than 1 hour, peak 30 minutes to 2 hours, duration 4–6 hours
- Rectal: onset slow, peak 1–2 hours, duration 3–4 hours
- Take crushed or whole with full glass of water
- Can give with food or milk to decrease GI upset
- Signs of chronic poisoning: rapid, weak pulse; dyspnea; cold, clammy extremities
- Signs of chronic overdose: bleeding, bruising, malaise, fever, sore throat, anorexia, jaundice
- OTC; Preg Cat B

• •

Side Effects

Nausea, vomiting Dyspnea GI bleeding
Rash Melena
Angioedema Tinnitus

Nursing Considerations

- Management of mild to moderate pain or fever, transient ischemic attacks, prophylaxis of MI, ischemic stroke, angina
- PO: onset 15–30 minutes, peak 1–2 hours, duration 4–6 hours
- Rectal: onset slow, 20%–60% absorbed if retained 2–4 hours
- With long-term use, check for liver damage: dark urine, clay-colored stools, yellowing of skin and sclera, itching, abdominal pain, fever, diarrhea
- For arthritis, give 30 minutes before exercise; may take 2 weeks before full effect is felt
- Discard tablets if vinegar-like smell
- Do not give to children or teens with flulike symptoms or chicken-pox; Reye syndrome may develop
- OTC; Preg Cat C

CELECOXIB
(sel-eh-<u>cox</u>-ib)

(Celebrex)

IBUPROFEN
(eye-byoo-<u>proe</u>-fen)

(Advil, Motrin IB)

Side Effects

Fatigue
Anxiety, depression,
nervousness
Nausea, vomiting, anorexia,
dry mouth, constipation
Angioedema

Hives
Dyspnea
Back pain
Tachycardia
Jaundice
Dysuria

Nursing Considerations

- Management of acute, chronic arthritis pain and primary
  dysmenorrheal pain relief within 60 minutes
- Onset: 24–48 hours, duration 12–24 hours
- Can take without regard to meals
- Increasing doses do not appear to increase effectiveness
- Do not take if allergic to sulfonamides, aspirin, or NSAIDs
- Rx; Preg Cat C for first and second trimester; Preg Cat D for
  third trimester

• •

Side Effects

Headache	Dizziness	GI bleeding
Tinnitus	Blood dyscrasias	
Nausea, anorexia	Constipation	

Nursing Considerations

- Treatment of rheumatoid arthritis, osteoarthritis, primary
  dysmenorrhea, gout, dental pain, musculoskeletal disorders, fever
- Onset: 30 minutes, peak 1–2 hours
- Contact clinician if ringing or roaring in ears, which may
  indicate toxicity
- Contact clinician if changes in urinary pattern, increased weight,
  edema, increased pain in joints, fever, or blood in urine, which may
  indicate kidney damage
- Use sunscreen to prevent photosensitivity
- Avoid use with ASA, NSAIDs, and alcohol, which may precipitate
  GI bleeding
- Avoid use with anticoagulants
- May have an increased risk of MI or stroke
- OTC, Rx; Preg Cat B

NAPROXEN
(na-<u>prox</u>-en)

(Aleve [OTC], Anaprox, Anaprox DS, Naprelan, EC-Naprosyn, Naprosyn)

• •

CODEINE
(<u>koe</u>-deen)

Side Effects

GI bleeding

Blood dyscrasias

Tinnitus

Headache

Insomnia

Vision changes

Rash

Angioedema

Jaundice

Tachycardia

Back pain

Nausea

Nursing Considerations

- Management of mild to moderate pain
- Treatment of rheumatoid, juvenile, and gouty arthritis; osteoarthritis; primary dysmenorrhea
- Patients with asthma, ASA hypersensitivity, or nasal polyps have increased risk of hypersensitivity
- Contact clinician if blurred vision or ringing or roaring in ears, which may indicate toxicity
- Contact clinician if black stools, flulike symptoms
- Contact clinician if changes in urinary pattern, increased weight, edema, increased pain in joints, fever, or blood in urine, which may indicate kidney damage
- Avoid use with ASA, steroids, and alcohol
- May increase risk of MI or stroke
- OTC, Rx; Preg Cat B

• •

Side Effects

Drowsiness, sedation

Nausea, vomiting, anorexia

Respiratory depression

Constipation

Orthostatic hypotension

Dysuria

Hives

Dyspnea

Syncope

Angioedema

Seizures

Nursing Considerations

- Treatment of moderate to severe pain, nonproductive cough
- PO: onset 30–45 minutes, peak 60–120 minutes, duration 4–6 hours
- IM/subQ: onset 10–30 minutes, peak 30–60 minutes, duration 4–6 hours
- Do not give if respirations are less than 12 per minute
- Avoid use with alcohol, CNS depressants
- Withdrawal symptoms may occur: nausea, vomiting, cramps, fever, faintness, anorexia
- Physical dependency may result from long-term use
- Rx C-II, III, IV, V (depends on route); Preg Cat C

HYDROCODONE BITARTRATE & ACETAMINOPHEN
(hi-dro-<u>ko</u>-doughne)

(Lortab, Vicodin)

• •

HYDROMORPHONE
(hye-droe-<u>mor</u>-fone)

(Dilaudid)

Side Effects

Dizziness

Drowsiness

Constipation

Nausea

Vomiting

Respiratory depression

Sedation

Impairment of mental and
physical performance

Rash

Pruritus

Nursing Considerations

- Used for relief of moderate to moderately severe pain
- Use with CNS depressants and/or alcohol may result in addictive CNS depression
- May be habit-forming
- Avoid alcohol during treatment
- Use with caution in patients with pulmonary considerations
- Rx C-III; Preg Cat C

• •

Side Effects

Drowsiness, sedation

Nausea, vomiting, anorexia

Respiratory depression

Constipation, cramps

Orthostatic hypotension

Confusion, headache

Rash

Nursing Considerations

- Treatment of moderate to severe pain, nonproductive cough
- PO: onset 15–30 minutes, peak 30–60 minutes, duration 4–6 hours
- IM: onset 15 minutes, peak 30–60 minutes, duration 4–5 hours
- IV: onset 10–15 minutes, peak 15–30 minutes, duration 2–3 hours
- subQ: onset 15 minutes, peak 30–90 minutes, duration 4 hours
- Rectal: duration 6–8 hours
- Do not give if respirations are less than 12 per minute
- Avoid use with alcohol, CNS depressants
- Withdrawal symptoms may occur: nausea, vomiting, cramps, fever, faintness, anorexia
- Physical dependency may result from long-term use
- Elderly patients may require lower doses
- Rx C-II; Preg Cat C

MEPERIDINE
(me-<u>per</u>-i-deen)

(Demerol)

• •

METHADONE
(<u>meth</u>-a-doan)

(Dolophine, Methadose)

Side Effects

Drowsiness, sedation	Orthostatic hypotension	Diaphoresis
Respiratory depression	Confusion, headache	Urticaria
Euphoria	Bradycardia	

Nursing Considerations

- Management of moderate to severe pain, pre-op sedation, post-op, and OB analgesia
- PO: onset 10–15 minutes, peak 30–60 minutes, duration 2–4 hours (usually 3)
- IM: onset 10–15 minutes, peak 30–50 minutes, duration 2–4 hours (usually 3)
- IV: onset less than 5 minutes, peak 5–7 minutes, duration 2–4 hours (usually 3)
- subQ: onset 10–15 minutes, peak 30–50 minutes, duration 2–4 hours (usually 3)
- Do not give if respirations are less than 12 per minute
- Avoid use with alcohol, CNS depressants
- Withdrawal symptoms may occur: nausea, vomiting, cramps, fever, faintness, anorexia
- Physical dependency may result from long-term use
- Do not co-infuse with barbiturates, aminophylline, heparin, morphine, methicillin, phenytoin, sodium bicarbonate, sulfadiazine, or sulfisoxazole
- Rx C-II; Preg Cat C

• •

Side Effects

Drowsiness, sedation	Orthostatic hypotension	Agitation
Nausea, vomiting, anorexia	Confusion, headache	Diaphoresis
Respiratory depression	Rash	Hypokalemia
Constipation, cramps	Arrhythmias	Pulmonary edema
	Syncope	

Nursing Considerations

- Relief of pain, detoxification/maintenance of narcotic addiction
- PO: onset 30–60 minutes, peak 30–60 minutes, duration 4–6 hours (with continuous dosing, duration of action may increase to 22 to 48 hours)
- IM: onset 10–20 minutes, peak 60–120 minutes, duration 4–5 hours (with continuous dosing, duration of action may increase to 22 to 48 hours)
- IV: onset peak 15–30 minutes, duration 3–4 hours
- Do not give if respirations are less than 12 per minute
- Avoid use with alcohol, CNS depressants
- Withdrawal symptoms may occur: nausea, vomiting, cramps, fever, faintness, anorexia
- Physical dependency may result from long-term use
- Rx C-II; Preg Cat C

MORPHINE

(<u>mor</u>-feen)

**(Astramorph PF, Avinza, Duramorph,
Infumorph, Kadian, MS Contin)**

• •

OXYCODONE

(ox-i-<u>koe</u>-done)

**(OxyContin; with aspirin Percodan,
with acetaminophen Percocet)**

Side Effects

Respiratory depression	Euphoria	Bradycardia
Sedation	Orthostatic hypotension	Diaphoresis
		Urticaria

Nursing Considerations

- Management of severe pain
- Continuous dosing is more effective than prn; may be given by patient controlled analgesia (PCA)
- PO: onset 15–60 minutes, peak 30–60 minutes, duration 3–6 hours
- IM: onset 10–15 minutes, peak 30–50 minutes, duration 2–4 hours (usually 3)
- IV: onset less than 5 minutes, peak 18 minutes, duration 3–6 hours
- subQ: onset 10–15 minutes, peak 30–50 minutes, duration 2–4 hours (usually 3)
- Withdrawal symptoms may occur: nausea, vomiting, cramps, fever, faintness, anorexia
- Physical dependency may result from long-term use
- Monitor for increased respiratory and CSN depression when given with cimetidine, clomipramine, nortriptyline, or amitriptyline
- Rx C-II; Preg Cat C

• •

Side Effects

Drowsiness, sedation	Rash
Nausea, vomiting, anorexia	Euphoria
Respiratory depression	Urinary retention
Constipation, cramps	Orthostatic hypotension
Confusion, headache	

Nursing Considerations

- Management of moderate to severe pain
- PO: peak 30–60 minutes, duration 4–6 hours
- Controlled-release: peak 3–4 minutes, duration 12 hours
- Do not give if respirations are less than 12 per minute
- Avoid use with alcohol, CNS depressants
- Withdrawal symptoms may occur: nausea, vomiting, cramps, fever, faintness, anorexia
- Physical dependency may result from long-term use
- Rx C-II; Preg Cat B (controlled-release); Preg Cat C (Percocet)

PROPOXYPHENE
(proe-<u>pox</u>-i-feen)

**(Darvon, Darvocet-N [propoxyphene
with acetaminophen])**

• •

HEPARIN
(<u>hep</u>-a-rin)

Side Effects

Drowsiness, sedation
Nausea, vomiting, anorexia
Respiratory depression
Constipation, cramps

Orthostatic hypotension
Confusion, headache
Rash
Hallucinations

Nursing Considerations

- Management of mild to moderate pain
- PO: onset 30–60 minutes, peak 120 minutes, duration 4–6 hours
- Low schedule rating for misuse potential, addiction liability
- Do not use in patients with suicidal tendencies
- Avoid use with alcohol, CNS depressants
- Withdrawal symptoms may occur: nausea, vomiting, cramps, fever, faintness, anorexia
- Physical dependency may result from long-term use with high doses
- Rx C-IV; Preg Cat C

· ·

Side Effects

Can produce hemorrhage from
  any body site (10%)
Tissue irritation/
  pain at injection site

Anemia
Thrombocytopenia
Fever

Nursing Considerations

- Prophylaxis and treatment of thromboembolic disorders in very low doses (10–100 units) to maintain patency of IV catheters (heparin flush)
- Therapeutic PTT @ 1.5–2.5 times the control without signs of hemorrhage
- IV: peak 5 minutes, duration 2–6 hours (give over 1 minute)
- Injection: give deep subQ; never IM (danger of hematoma), onset 20–60 minutes, duration 8–12 hours
- Antidote: protamine sulfate within 30 minutes
- Signs of hemorrhage: bleeding gums, epistaxis (nosebleed) , unusual bleeding, black or tarry stools, hematuria, fall in hematocrit or blood pressure, guaiac-positive stools
- Avoid ASA-containing products and NSAIDs
- Wear medical information tag
- Abrupt withdrawal may precipitate increased coagulability
- Rx; Preg Cat C

Anticoagulants
Anticoagulants

WARFARIN
(<u>war</u>-far-in)

(Coumadin, Jantoven)

. . . .

Anticonvulsants
Anticonvulsants

CARBAMAZEPINE
(kar-ba-<u>maz</u>-e-peen)

**(Carbatrol, Epitol, Equetro,
Tegretol, Tegretol XR)**

Side Effects

Hemorrhage
Diarrhea
Rash
Fever
Angina syndrome

Syncope
Anemia
Dermatitis
Jaundice

Elevated liver
enzymes
Anaphylactic
reactions

Nursing Considerations

- Management of pulmonary emboli, deep vein thrombosis, MI, atrial dysrhythmias, postcardiac valve replacement
- Therapeutic PT @ 1.5–2.5 times the control, INR @ 2.0–3.0
- Onset: 12–24 hours, peak 1.5 to 3 days; duration 3 to 5 days
- Avoid foods high in vitamin K: many green leafy vegetables
- Do not interchange brands; potencies may not be equivalent
- Do not take any drug or herb without physician approval—may change effect
- Avoid ASA-containing products and NSAIDs
- Oral anticoagulants may cause red-orange discoloration of alkaline urine, interfering with some lab tests
- Wear medical information tag
- Rx; Preg Cat X

• •

Side Effects

Myelosuppression
Dizziness, drowsiness
Ataxia
Diplopia, rash
Photosensitivity

Depression
Nausea
Vomiting
Dyspepsia
Apastic anemia

Stevens-Johnson
syndrome
Suicide attempts in
bipolar patients

Nursing Considerations

- Management of seizures, trigeminal neuralgia, diabetic neuropathy
- Avoid driving and other activities requiring alertness the first 3 days
- Monitor blood levels, CBC regularly, esp. during first 2 months; periodic eye exams
- Take with food or milk to decrease GI upset; tablets (nonextended-release) may be crushed, extended-release capsules may be opened and mixed with juice or soft food (no grapefruit products)
- Urine may turn pink to brown
- Avoid abrupt withdrawal; discontinue gradually
- Avoid use with alcohol, CNS depressants
- Inform physician before taking any new medication or herbal medication
- Rx; Preg Cat D

DIVALPROEX SODIUM
(dye-<u>val</u>-proe-ex)

(Depakote, Depakote ER)

• •

GABAPENTIN
(ga-ba-<u>pen</u>-tin)

(Gabarone, Neurontin)

Side Effects

Sedation, drowsiness, dizziness
Mental status and behavioral changes
Nausea, vomiting, constipation, diarrhea

Heartburn
Prolonged bleeding time
Hepatotoxicity
Teratogenicity
Pancreatitis
Thrombocytopenia

Headache
Diplopia
Tremor
Alopecia
Multiorgan hypersensitivity

Nursing Considerations

- Management of seizures, manic episodes assoc. with bipolar disorder (delayed-release only), migraine prophylaxis (delayed- and extended-release only)
- Take with or immediately after meals to lessen GI upset; swallow whole
- Avoid abrupt withdrawal after long-term use; discontinue gradually to prevent convulsions
- Monitor blood levels, platelets, bleeding time, and liver function tests
- Delayed-release products: peak blood level 3–5 hours, duration 12–24 hours
- Extended-release products: onset 2–4 days, peak blood level 7–14 hours, duration 24 hours
- Wear medical information tag
- Rx; Preg Cat D

• •

Side Effects

Drowsiness
Ataxia
Diplopia
Rhinitis

Constipation
Memory problems
Uncontrolled shaking

Back or joint pain
Edema
Flulike symptoms
Seizures

Nursing Considerations

- Used for management of seizures and postherpetic neuralgia, diabetic neuropathy
- Do not take within 2 hours of antacid use
- Avoid abrupt withdrawal after long-term use; discontinue gradually over a week to prevent convulsions
- Give without regard to meals; can open capsules and put in juice or applesauce
- Do not crush or chew capsules
- Use caution with hazardous activities
- Wear medical information tag
- Rx; Preg Cat C

LAMOTRIGINE
(la-<u>moe</u>-tri-jeen)

(Lamictal)

• •

PHENOBARBITAL
(fee-noe-<u>bar</u>-bi-tal)

(Luminal)

Side Effects

Ataxia, dizziness
Headache
Nausea, vomiting, anorexia
Diplopia, blurred vision
Abdominal pain, dysmenorrhea

Loss of coordination
Mood changes
Irritability
Insomnia
Depression

Nursing Considerations

- Used for management of seizures, abnormal mood disorders
- In pediatric patients, stop at first sign of rash; all patients should notify clinician of rashes
- Take divided doses with meals or just after to decrease adverse effects
- Use caution with hazardous activities until stabilized
- Avoid abrupt withdrawal; stop gradually to prevent increase in frequency of seizures
- Wear medical information tag
- Rx; Preg Cat C

• •

Side Effects

Drowsiness, lethargy, rash
GI upset
Initially constricts pupils
Respiratory depression
Ataxia

Nightmares
Unusual bleeding
Dyspnea
Dysphagia
Excitement in children

Nursing Considerations

- Management of epilepsy, febrile seizures in children, sedation, insomnia
- IV: slow rate—resuscitation equipment should be available
- IM: inject deep into large muscle mass to prevent tissue sloughing, can give subQ, onset 10–30 minutes
- PO: onset 20–60 minutes, peak 8–12 hours, duration 6–10 hours
- Use caution with hazardous activities until stabilized; drowsiness usually diminishes after initial weeks of therapy
- Nystagmus may indicate early toxicity
- Long-term use withdrawal symptoms: vomiting, sweating, abdomen/muscle cramps, tremors, and possibly convulsions
- Vitamin D supplements are indicated for long-term use
- Rx C-IV; Preg Cat D

PHENYTOIN
(<u>fen</u>-i-toyn)
(Dilantin)

• •

PREGABALIN
(pre-<u>gab</u>-a-lin)
(Lyrica)

Side Effects

Drowsiness, ataxia
Nystagmus
Blurred vision
Hirsutism

Lethargy
GI upset
Gingival
Hypertrophy

Suicidal behavior
Skin rash

Nursing Considerations

- Management of seizures, migraines, trigeminal neuralgia, Bell's palsy
- PO: take divided doses, with or immediately after meals, to decrease adverse effects
- May color urine and sweat pink/red/brown
- May cause increase in blood sugar
- IV administration may lead to cardiac arrest—have resuscitation equipment available; never mix in IV with any other drug or dextrose
- Avoid abrupt withdrawal to prevent convulsions
- Do not use antacids or antidiarrheals within 2 hours of med
- Use caution with hazardous activities until stabilized
- Folic acid supplements are indicated for long-term use
- Wear medical information tag
- Rx; Preg Cat D

• •

Side Effects

Dizziness, tiredness, weakness
Headache
Nausea, vomiting, constipation
Flatulence, bloating
Mental status and behavioral changes
Anxiety

Lack of coordination, loss of balance, unsteadiness
Uncontrollable shaking or jerking of a part of the body, muscle twitching
Increased appetite, weight gain

Swelling of the arms, hands, feet, ankles, or lower legs
Back pain
Infection
Angioedema
Neuropathy

Nursing Considerations

- Treatment for neuropathic pain, diabetic pain, pain after shingles, fibromyalgia, and partial onset seizures in adults with epilepsy who already take one or more drugs for seizures
- Take around the same time every day, two to three times daily; full therapeutic effects may require 4 weeks
- Avoid abrupt withdrawal after long-term use; discontinue gradually
- Avoid use with alcohol
- Use caution in potentially hazardous activities
- May increase the risk of suicidal thoughts or behavior
- Rx; Preg Cat C

TOPIRAMATE
(toh-<u>pire</u>-ah-mate)

(Topamax, Topiragen)

· ·

VALPROATE
(val-<u>proe</u>-ate)

(Depacon)

Side Effects

Dizziness, drowsiness, fatigue
Impaired concentration/memory
Nervousness, speech problems
Nausea, weight loss
Vision problems

Ataxia
Photosensitivity
Behavior problems,
  mood problems
Anorexia

Nursing Considerations

- Used for management of seizures, prophylaxis of migraine headache, cluster headache, bulimia
- Give without regard to meals; can open capsules and put in juice or applesauce
- Avoid abrupt withdrawal after long-term use; discontinue gradually to prevent seizures and status epilepticus
- Use caution with hazardous activities until stabilized
- Increase fluid intake to prevent formation of kidney stones
- Stop drug immediately if eye problems; could lead to permanent loss of vision
- Use sunscreen and protective clothing to prevent photosensitivity
- Wear medical information tag
- Rx; Preg Cat C

• •

Side Effects

Sedation, drowsiness, dizziness
Mental status and behavioral
  changes
Nausea, vomiting, constipation,
  diarrhea, heartburn

Prolonged bleeding time
Hepatotoxicity
Teratogenicity
Pancreatitis

Nursing Considerations

- Used for management of seizures, manic episodes associated with bipolar disorders, prevent migraines
- Avoid abrupt withdrawal after long-term use; discontinue gradually to prevent convulsions
- May be given with food to decrease GI irritation
- Monitor blood levels, platelets, bleeding time, and liver function tests
- Onset of anticonvulsant effect: 2–4 days, peak blood level at end of infusion, duration 6–24 hours
- Rx; Preg Cat D

VALPROIC ACID
(val-<u>proe</u>-ic)

(Depakene, Myproic Acid)

· ·

AMIKACIN, GENTAMICIN, TOBRAMYCIN
(am-i-<u>kay</u>-sin, jen-ta-<u>mye</u>-sin,
toe-bra-<u>mye</u>-sin)

(Amikin, Garamycin, Tobrex)

Side Effects

Sedation, drowsiness, dizziness

Mental status and behavioral changes

Nausea, vomiting, constipation, diarrhea, heartburn

Prolonged bleeding time

Hepatotoxicity

Teratogenicity

Pancreatitis

Nursing Considerations

- Used for management of seizures, mania, prevent migraine headaches
- Take with or immediately after meals to lessen GI upset
- Swallow capsules whole (no crushing, chewing)
- Avoid abrupt withdrawal after long-term use; discontinue gradually to prevent convulsions
- Monitor blood levels, platelets, bleeding time, and liver function tests
- Onset: 2–4 days, peak blood level of syrup 15–120 minutes, of capsules 1–4 hours, duration 6–24 hours (varies with age)
- Wear medical information tag
- Rx; Preg Cat D

• •

Side Effects

Use during pregnancy can result in bilateral congenital deafness

Ototoxicity cranial nerve VIII

Nephrotoxicity

Allergic reaction: fever, difficulty breathing, rash

Vertigo, tinnitus

Nursing Considerations

- Treatment of severe systemic infections of CNS, respiratory, GI, urinary tract, bone, skin, soft tissues, acute PID
- IV over 30 minutes to 1 hour; IM by deep, slow injection, never subQ
- Careful monitoring of blood levels
- Check peak—2 hours after med given
- Check trough—at time of dose/prior to med
- Monitor for signs of superinfection (diarrhea, URI, coated tongue)
- Immediately report hearing or balance problems
- Encourage fluids to 8–10 glasses/day
- Rx; Preg Cat D

AMPHOTERICIN B
(am-foe-<u>ter</u>-i-sin)

(Abelcet, Amphotec, Fungizone)

. . . .

FLUCONAZOLE
(flew-<u>kon</u>-uh-zol)

(Diflucan)

Side Effects

Blood, kidney, heart, liver abnormalities

GI upset

Hypokalemia-induced muscle pain

CNS disturbances, inefficient hearing

Skin irritation and thrombosis if IV infiltrates

Rash

Fever

Malaise

Hypotension

Headache

Nephrotoxicity

Nursing Considerations

- Do not mix with other drugs
- Treatment of histoplasmosis, skin infections, septicemia, meningitis in HIV patients
- Monitor vital signs; report fever or change in function, especially nervous system
- Check for hypokalemia
- Meticulous care and observation of injection site
- Potential benefits must be balanced against serious side effects
- Rx; Preg Cat B

• •

Side Effects

Nausea

Headache

Abdominal pain

Diarrhea

Taste distortion

Nursing Considerations

- Used to treat vaginal, esophageal, or systemic candidiasis; cryptococcal meningitis
- Prothrombin time is increased after warfarin usage
- Take missed dose as soon as noticed, but do not double dose
- Reduces metabolism of tolbutamide, glyburide, and glipizide,
- Glucose levels should be monitored, especially in diabetics
- Rx; Preg Cat C

HYDROXYCHLOROQUINE
(hye-drox-ee-<u>klor</u>-oh-kwin)

(Plaquenil)

· ·

QUININE SULFATE
(<u>kwye</u>-nine)

Side Effects

Eye disturbances
Nausea, vomiting
Anorexia

Rash
Headache
Loss of hair

Nursing Considerations

- Management of malaria, lupus erythematosus, rheumatoid arthritis
- Peak 1–2 hours
- Take at the same time each day to maintain blood level
- Give with meats to decrease GI distress
- For malaria, prophylaxis should be started 2 weeks before exposure and continue for 4–6 weeks after leaving exposure area
- Rx; Preg Cat C

• •

Side Effects

Eye disturbances
Nausea, vomiting

Anorexia

Nursing Considerations

- Treatment of malaria, nocturnal leg cramps
- Peak 1–3 hours
- Take at the same time each day to maintain blood level
- Avoid OTC cold meds, tonic water
- May increase digoxin levels
- OTC, Rx; Preg Cat X

METRONIDAZOLE
(me-troe-<u>nye</u>-da-zole)

(Flagyl, Flagyl ER)

• •

ISONIAZID
(eye-soe-<u>nye</u>-a-zid)

(INH)

Side Effects

Headache
Dizziness
Nausea, vomiting, diarrhea

Abdominal cramps
Metallic taste

Nursing Considerations

- Treatment of a wide variety of infections, including trichomoniasis and giardiasis
- IV: immediate onset, PO: peak 1–2 hours
- Urine may turn dark reddish-brown
- Avoid hazardous activities
- Treatment of both partners is necessary in trichomoniasis
- Do not drink alcohol or preparations containing alcohol during and 48 hours after use, disulfiram-like reaction can occur
- Rx; Preg Cat B

• •

Side Effects

Peripheral neuropathy

Liver damage

Nursing Considerations

- Prevention and treatment of TB
- PO/IM: onset rapid, peak 1–2 hours, duration up to 24 hours
- Contact clinician if signs of hepatitis: yellow eyes and skin, nausea, vomiting, anorexia, dark urine, unusual tiredness, or weakness
- Contact clinician if signs of peripheral neuropathy: numbness, tingling, or weakness
- Monitor liver tests
- Rx; Preg Cat C

ACYCLOVIR
(ay-<u>sye</u>-kloe-ver)

(Zovirax)

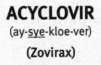

OSELTAMIVIR PHOSPHATE
(oh-sul-<u>tamm</u>-eh-vere)

(Tamiflu)

Side Effects

Headache
Blood dyscrasias

Nausea, vomiting,
  diarrhea

Nursing Considerations

- Treatment of herpes, varicella
- IV: onset immediate, peak immediate
- PO: absorbed minimally, onset unknown, peak 90 minutes
- Do not break, crush, or chew capsules
- PO: take without regard to meals with a full glass of water
- If dose is missed, take as soon as remembered, up to 1 hour before next dose
- Contact clinician if sore throat, fever and fatigue; could be signs of superinfection
- May cause acute renal failure; monitor renal function
- Thrombocytopenic purpura
- Rx; Preg Cat B

• •

Side Effects

Nausea
Vomiting
Dizziness

Headache
Fatigue
Cough

Nursing Considerations

- Used as prophylaxis in adults for influenza, including avian bird flu
- Used to treat uncomplicated acute flu symptoms in patients that are symptomatic for 2 days or less
- Should not be used as a substitute for influenza vaccinations
- May be taken without regard to meals
- Rx; Preg Cat C

VALACYCLOVIR HCL
(val-uh-<u>sy</u>-klo-veer)

(Valtrex)

· ·

ZIDOVUDINE
(zye-<u>doe</u>-vue-deen)

(AZT, Retrovir)

Side Effects

Nausea, vomiting, diarrhea
Abdominal cramps
Headache

Rash
Fatigue
Dizziness

Nursing Considerations

- For the treatment of genital herpes
- Used to treat herpes zoster (shingles)
- Used to treat herpes labialis (cold sores)
- Patients should drink plenty of fluids during treatment
- Avoid sexual contact when lesions are visible
- Use with caution in pregnancy and nursing mothers
- Rx; Preg Cat B

• •

Side Effects

Fever, headache, malaise
Nausea, vomiting, diarrhea
Dizziness
Insomnia

Dyspepsia
Anorexia
Rash

Nursing Considerations

- Management of HIV infections and prevention of HIV following needlestick
- GI upset and insomnia resolve after 3–4 weeks
- PO: peak 30–90 minutes
- Rx; Preg Cat C

CEFADROXIL
(sef-a-<u>drox</u>-ill)

(Duricef)

• •

CEPHALEXIN
(sef-a-<u>lex</u>-in)

(Keflex)

Side Effects

Diarrhea   Rash
Angioedema

Nursing Considerations

- Treatment of upper and lower respiratory tract, urinary tract, and skin infections, otitis media, tonsillitis, and UTIs
- Peak 60–90 minutes, duration 12–24 hours
- Take for 10–14 days to prevent superinfection
- Possible cross-allergy to penicillin
- May alter results (false positive) of urine glucose
- Rx; Preg Cat B

• •

Side Effects

Diarrhea   Rash
Anaphylaxis   Headache
Nausea

Nursing Considerations

- Treatment of upper and lower respiratory tract, urinary tract, and skin infections, bone infections, otitis media
- Peak 1 hour, duration usually 6 hours, but may be up to 12 hours with decreased renal function
- Take for 10–14 days to prevent superinfection
- Possible cross-allergy to penicillin
- May cause false positive of urine glucose
- Rx; Preg Cat B

CEPHRADINE

(<u>sef</u>-ra-deen)

(Velosef)

• •

CEFACLOR

(<u>sef</u>-a-klor)

(Ceclor, Ceclor CD)

Side Effects

Diarrhea   Dizziness
Rash

Nursing Considerations

- Treatment of serious respiratory tract and skin infections, otitis media, and UTIs
- Peak 1–2 hours, duration usually 6 hours, but may be up to 12 hours with decreased renal function
- Take for 10–14 days to prevent superinfection
- May cause false positive of urine glucose; use only Clinistix, Diastix, or Tes-Tape for testing
- Rx; Preg Cat B

● ●

Side Effects

Diarrhea

Nursing Considerations

- Treatment of respiratory tract, urinary tract, bone, joint, and skin infections, otitis media
- Peak 30–60 minutes, extended-release peak 1.5–2.5 hours
- Take for 10–14 days to prevent superinfection
- May cause false positive in urine glucose
- Rx; Preg Cat B

CEFOTETAN
(<u>sef</u>-oh-tee-tan)

• •

CEFOXITIN
(se-<u>fox</u>-i-tin)

(Mefoxin)

Side Effects

Diarrhea   Nausea

Rash

Nursing Considerations

- Treatment of respiratory tract, urinary tract, bone, joint, and skin infections, GYN and gonococcal infections, intra-abdominal infections
- IM/IV: peak 1.5–3 hours or at end of infusion
- Avoid alcohol
- May cause falsely elevated serum or urine creatinine values
- Rx; Preg Cat B

• •

Side Effects

Diarrhea

Rash

Nursing Considerations

- Treatment of respiratory tract, urinary tract, bone and skin infections, GYN and gonococcal infections, peritonitis, septicemia
- IM: peak 20–30 minutes
- IV: peak at end of infusion
- Take for 10–14 days to prevent superinfection
- Avoid alcohol
- Eat yogurt or buttermilk to maintain intestinal flora
- May cause false positive urine glucose
- Rx; Preg Cat B

CEFPROZIL
(sef-<u>proe</u>-zill)

(Cefzil)

• •

CEFUROXIME
(sef-yoor-<u>ox</u>-eem)

(Ceftin, Zinacef)

Side Effects
Diarrhea
Rash

Nursing Considerations
- Treatment of pharyngitis/tonsillitis, otitis media, secondary bacterial infection of acute bronchitis, and acute bacterial exacerbation of chronic bronchitis, acute sinusitis
- Peak 90 minutes
- Take for 10–14 days to prevent superinfection
- May cause false positive Coombs test
- May cause elevated levels in ALT, AST
- May cause false positive urine glucose
- Rx; Preg Cat B

• •

Side Effects
Diarrhea
Rash

Nursing Considerations
- Treatment of respiratory tract, urinary tract, bone and skin infections, gonococcal infections, meningitis, septicemia
- Take for 10–14 days to prevent superinfection
- May cause increased BUN and serum creatine
- May cause false positive urine glucose
- Rx; Preg Cat B

CEFDINIR
(<u>sef</u>-dih-ner)

(Omnicef)

. . . .

CEFEPIME
(<u>sef</u>-e-peem)

(Maxipime)

Side Effects

Nausea, vomiting, diarrhea   Headache
Anorexia   Vaginal yeast infection
Rash

Nursing Considerations

- Treatment of acute exacerbations of chronic bronchitis, sinusitis, pharyngitis, otitis media, tonsillitis, skin infections
- Take for 10–14 days to prevent superinfection
- Do not give antacids or iron supplements within 2 hours
- May cause false positive for urine ketones or glucose
- May cause increased GGT
- Rx; Preg Cat B

• •

Side Effects

Nausea, vomiting, diarrhea   Rash
Anorexia   Headache
Elevated liver function tests

Nursing Considerations

- Treatment of respiratory tract, urinary, and skin infections
- IV: peak 30 minutes
- IM: peak 2 hours
- May cause false positive Coombs test
- May cause false positive for urine glucose
- Rx; Preg Cat B

CEFOTAXIME
(sef-oh-<u>taks</u>-eem)

(Claforan)

• •

CEFPODOXIME
(sef-poe-<u>docks</u>-eem)

(Vantin)

Side Effects

Nausea, vomiting, diarrhea   Rash
Anorexia

Nursing Considerations

- Treatment of respiratory tract, intra-abdominal/GYN infections, gonococcal infections, meningitis, septicemia, bacteremia
- IV: onset 5 minutes
- IM: onset 30 minutes
- Monitor for superinfection
- Yogurt or buttermilk may help maintain normal intestinal flora
- Monitor I & O
- May cause falsely elevated serum or urine creatinine
- Rx; Preg Cat B

• •

Side Effects

Nausea, vomiting, diarrhea   Urticaria
Anorexia   Cough

Nursing Considerations

- Treatment of respiratory tract, urinary tract, and skin infections, otitis media, and STD infections
- Take for 10–14 days to prevent superinfection
- Give 1 or 2 hours after antacid
- Give with food to enhance absorption
- Rx; Preg Cat B

CIPROFLOXACIN
(sip-ro-<u>flocks</u>-a-sin)

(Cipro)

• •

LEVOFLOXACIN
(lee-voe-<u>flocks</u>-a-sin)

(Levaquin)

Side Effects

Seizures
Nausea, vomiting, diarrhea,
    abd. distress, flatulence
Rash

Photosensitivity
Tendon rupture, muscle tear
CNS side effects

Nursing Considerations

- Treatment of infection caused by *E. coli* and other bacteria, chronic bacterial prostatitis, acute sinusitis, postexposure inhalation anthrax
- Contraindicated in children less than 18 years of age
- Take 2 hours pc or 2 hours before an antacid or iron preparation
- Take at equal intervals around the clock
- Avoid caffeine
- Encourage fluids to 8–10 glasses/day
- May cause false positive in opiate screening tests
- Do not infuse with other medications
- Rx; Preg Cat C

• •

Side Effects

Headache, nausea, vomiting,
    diarrhea, constipation
Stomach pain
Dizziness, heartburn
Vaginal itching and/or discharge
Tendon rupture or tendinitis

Irritation, pain, tenderness,
    redness, warmth, or swelling
    at the injection spot
Seizures, confusion, rash
Hallucination, paranoia
Angioedema

Nursing Considerations

- Treatment of infections such as endocarditis, tuberculosis, anthrax, pneumonia, chronic bronchitis, and infections involving the sinus, urinary tract, kidney, prostate, or skin
- Infused injection over 60–90 minutes, once every 24 hours
- Teach patient to avoid sunlamps, tanning beds, and to limit time in sun
- Avoid activities that require alertness or coordination
- Monitor for hepatotoxicity
- May increase risk of suicidal thoughts or behaviors
- Monitor blood sugar; may cause hypoglycemia or hyperglycemia
- Teach patient to notify physician immediately for change in heartbeat
- Rx; Preg Cat C

VANCOMYCIN
(van-koe-<u>my</u>-sin)

(Vancocin)

• •

CLINDAMYCIN HCL PHOSPHATE
(klin-da-<u>my</u>-sin)

(Cleocin HCl, Cleocin Phosphate for IM)

Side Effects

Liver damage
Nephrotoxicity

Tinnitus or hearing loss

Nursing Considerations

- Treatment of resistant staph infections, colitis, staph enterocolitis, endocarditis prophylaxis for dental procedures (used for *C. difficile*)
- PO: poor absorption
- IV: peak 5 minutes, duration 12–24 hours
- Give antihistamine if "red man syndrome": decreased blood pressure, flushing of face and neck
- Give at least 60 minutes (IV); do not infuse with other drugs
- Contact clinician if signs of superinfection: sore throat, fever, fatigue
- Rx; Preg Cat C

• •

Side Effects

Nausea, vomiting, diarrhea
Abdominal pain
Vaginitis

Rash
Jaundice

Nursing Considerations

- Treatment of infections caused by *Staphylococcus, Streptococcus,* and other organisms
- PO: peak 45 minutes, duration 6 hours
- IM: peak 3 hours, duration 8–12 hours
- May cause increase in AST, ALT, CPK
- Rx; Preg Cat B

AZITHROMYCIN
(ay-zi-thro-<u>my</u>-sin)

(Zithromax)

· ·

CLARITHROMYCIN
(klair-ith-row-<u>my</u>-sin)

(Biaxin, Biaxin XL)

Side Effects

Nausea, vomiting, diarrhea

Nursing Considerations

- Treatment of mild to moderate infections of the respiratory tract, skin, nongonococcal urethritis, cervicitis, acute pharyngitis/tonsillitis, community acquired pneumonia
- PO: rapid onset, peak 2.5–3.2 hours, duration 24 hours
- IV: rapid onset, peak end of infusion, duration 24 hours
- PO: don't take with antacids; can take with or without food
- Monitor for signs of superinfection (diarrhea, perineal itching, oral ulcers)
- If treated for nongonococcal urethritis or cervicitis, sexual partners also need treatment
- Rx; Preg Cat B

• •

Side Effects

Nausea	Dyspepsia
Taste abnormalities	Headache
Diarrhea	

Nursing Considerations

- Used for respiratory infections, pharyngitis/tonsillitis, sinusitis
- Treatment may be 7–14 days depending on organism and extent of infection
- Medication should be taken with food
- Be aware of possible increase in theophylline and carbamazepine levels
- Rx; Preg Cat C

ERYTHROMYCIN
(eh-rith-roe-<u>my</u>-sin)
(Ery-Tab, Erythrocin)

. . . .

AMOXICILLIN, AMPICILLIN, PENICILLIN
(ah-mox-ih-<u>sill</u>-in, am-pih-<u>sill</u>-in, pen-i-<u>sill</u>-in)
(Bicillin, DisperMox, Larotid, Moxatag, Omnipen, Wycillin)

Side Effects

Abdominal cramps
Pain at injection site
Nausea, vomiting, diarrhea

Rash
Anaphylaxis

Nursing Considerations

- Treatment of infections, including chlamydia, syphilis
- PO: give 1 hr ac/2 hr pc with full glass water (avoid citrus juice); some formulations can be given without regard to meals
- PO: onset 1 hour, peak up to 4 hours, duration 6–12 hours
- IV: onset rapid, peak end of infusion, duration 6–12 hours
- Take at equal intervals around the clock
- Can be used in patients with compromised renal function
- Monitor for signs of superinfection (diarrhea, perineal itching, oral ulcers)
- Rx; Preg Cat B

• •

Side Effects

Allergic reactions: fever, difficulty breathing, skin rash
Renal, hepatic, hematologic abnormalities

Nausea, vomiting, diarrhea

Nursing Considerations

- Treatment of respiratory infections, scarlet fever, otitis media, pneumonia, skin and soft tissue infections, gonorrhea
- Take careful history of penicillin reaction; observe for 20 minutes post IM injection
- PO for penicillin and ampicillin: take 1 hr ac or 2 hr pc to reduce gastric acid destruction of drug; not true for amoxicillin
- Take equally divided doses around the clock
- Continue medication for entire time prescribed, even if symptoms resolve
- Check for hypersensitivity to other drugs, especially cephalosporins
- Rx; Preg Cat B

SULFISOXAZOLE
(sul-fi-<u>sox</u>-a-zole)

• •

TRIMETHOPRIM-SULFAMETHOXAZOLE
(trye-<u>meth</u>-oh-prim-sul-fa-meth-<u>ox</u>-a-zole)

(Bactrim, Septra)

Side Effects

Headache
Nausea, vomiting, diarrhea
Allergic rash

Urinary crystallization
Photosensitivity

Nursing Considerations

- Treatment of urinary tract, systemic infections, chancroid, trachoma, toxoplasmosis, acute otitis media, malaria (adjunctive therapy), meningitis, eye infections
- PO: full glass water
- Monitor I & O, force fluids
- Rx; Preg Cat C

• •

Side Effects

Hypersensitivity reaction
Stop at first sign of skin rash
Blood dyscrasias

Photosensitivity
Nausea, vomiting, anorexia
Stomatitis, abdominal pain

Nursing Considerations

- Treatment of UTI, chancroid, acute otitis media, acute and chronic prostatitis, shigellosis, pneumonitis, chronic bronchitis, traveler's diarrhea
- PO: with full glass water; if upset stomach occurs, take with food
- PO: take at equal intervals around the clock
- IV solution must be given slowly over 60–90 minutes; flush lines at end of infusion to remove residual
- Never administer IM, rapidly IV, or by bolus injection
- Encourage fluids to 8–10 glasses/day
- Rx; Preg Cat C

DOXYCYCLINE HYCLATE
(dox-i-<u>sye</u>-kleen)

(Vibramycin, Vibra-Tabs)

· ·

MINOCYCLINE HCL
(mi-noe-<u>sye</u>-kleen)

(Minocin)

Side Effects

Photosensitivity
GI upset, diarrhea
Renal, hepatic, hematologic
  abnormalities

Dental discoloration of
  deciduous (baby) teeth

Nursing Considerations

- Treatment of syphilis, chlamydia, gonorrhea, malaria prophylaxis, chronic periodontitis, acne, anthrax
- Peak 1.5–4 hours
- If GI symptoms occur, administer with food EXCEPT milk products or other foods high in calcium (interferes with absorption)
- Take with full glass of water, do NOT take within 1 hour of bedtime or reclining
- Check patient's tongue for monilial infection
- Discard outdated prescriptions
- Avoid prolonged exposure to direct sunlight, UV light
- Avoid during tooth and early development periods (4th month prenatal to 8 years of age)
- Anticoagulant therapy may need to be adjusted
- Rx; Preg Cat D

• •

Side Effects

Photosensitivity
GI upset, diarrhea
Renal, hepatic, hematologic
  abnormalities

Dental discoloration of
  deciduous (baby) teeth

Nursing Considerations

- Treatment of chlamydia, periodontitis, acne, Rocky Mountain spotted fever, respiratory tract infections, meningitis
- Peak 2–3 hours
- If GI symptoms occur, administer with food EXCEPT milk products or other foods high in calcium (interferes with absorption)
- Take with full glass of water, do NOT take within 1 hour of bedtime
- Check patient's tongue for monilial infection
- Discard outdated prescriptions
- Avoid prolonged exposure to direct sunlight, UV light
- Avoid during tooth and early development periods (4th month prenatal to 8 years of age)
- Rx; Preg Cat D

HYDROCORTISONE
(hy-dro-<u>kor</u>-tih-sone)

(Cortef, Solu-Cortef)

· ·

METHYLPREDNISOLONE
(meth-ill-pred-<u>niss</u>-oh-lone)

(Medrol)

Side Effects

Depression

Flushing, sweating

Hypertension

Nausea, diarrhea

Hyperglycemia

Psychic derangements

Nursing Considerations

- Treatment of severe inflammation, septic shock, adrenal insufficiency, ulcerative colitis, collagen disorders
- Med masks signs of infection, so check for elevated temperature, WBC count
- PO: take with food, milk, antacids
- IM: give deep into gluteal UOQ, avoid deltoid, rotate sites, avoid subQ administration because it may damage tissue
- Monitor blood sugar in diabetes carefully
- Rectal: for colitis, retain med for 20 minutes, onset 3–5 days
- Wear medical information tag
- Do not mix with other medicines
- Rx; Preg Cat C

- -

Side Effects

Peptic ulcer/possible perforation

Hypertension and circulatory problems

Poor wound healing

Hyperglycemia

Psychic derangements

Nursing Considerations

- Treatment of severe inflammation, shock, adrenal insufficiency, management of acute spinal cord injury, collagen disorders
- PO: take with food, milk, antacids
- PO: peak 1–2 hours, duration 1.5 days
- IM: give deep into gluteal UOQ, avoid deltoid, rotate sites, avoid subQ administration because it may damage tissue
- IM: peak 4–8 days, duration 1–4 week
- Eat food high in protein, calcium, vitamin D; avoid sodium
- Contact clinician if anorexia, difficulty breathing, weakness, dizziness; symptoms may appear during periods of stress or trauma
- Contact clinician if black/tarry stools, slow wound healing, blurred vision, bruising/bleeding, weight gain, emotional changes
- Wear medical information tag
- Monitor patient weight, blood sugars
- Rx; Preg Cat C

PREDNISOLONE
(pred-<u>niss</u>-oh-lone)

(Delta-Cortef, Flo-Pred, Pred Forte, Prelone)

• •

PREDNISONE
(<u>pred</u>-ni-sone)

(Deltasone, Meticorten, Prednisone Intensol)

Side Effects

Depression

Hypertension, circulatory
  problems

Nausea, diarrhea

Abdominal distention

Nursing Considerations

- Treatment of severe inflammation, immunosuppression, neoplasms
- PO: take with food, milk, antacids
- PO: peak 1–2 hours, duration 3–36 hours
- IM: give deep into gluteal UOQ, avoid deltoid, rotate sites, avoid subQ administration because it may damage tissue
- IM: peak 1 hour, duration 4 weeks
- Eat food high in protein, calcium, vitamin D; avoid sodium
- Contact clinician if anorexia, difficulty breathing, weakness, dizziness; symptoms may appear during periods of stress or trauma
- Contact clinician if black/tarry stools, slow wound healing, blurred vision, bruising/bleeding, weight gain, emotional changes
- Wear medical information tag
- Rx; Preg Cat C

• •

Side Effects

Peptic ulcer/possible perforation

Depression

Hypertension, circulatory
  problems

Nausea, diarrhea

Abdominal distention

Hyperglycemia

Psychic derangements

Nursing Considerations

- Treatment of severe inflammation, immune suppression, neoplasms, multiple sclerosis, collagen disorders, dermatologic disorders, myasthenia gravis
- PO: take with food, milk, antacids
- PO: peak 1–2 hours, duration 1–1.5 days
- Eat food high in protein, calcium, vitamin D; avoid sodium
- Contact clinician if anorexia, difficulty breathing, weakness, dizziness; symptoms may appear during periods of stress or trauma
- Contact clinician if black/tarry stools, slow wound healing, blurred vision, bruising/bleeding, weight gain, emotional changes
- Excessive consumption of licorice can increase risk of hypokalemia
- Wear medical information tag
- Monitor blood sugar in diabetic patients
- Rx; Preg Cat C

NABUMETONE
(nay-<u>boom</u>-eh-tone)

• •

IBUPROFEN
(eye-byoo-<u>proe</u>-fen)

(Advil, Motrin IB)

Side Effects

Abdominal pain	Flatulence	Headache
Constipation	Tinnitus	Rash
Diarrhea	Edema	Gastritis

Nursing Considerations

- Used to manage symptoms of osteoarthritis and rheumatoid arthritis
- Take with food or milk
- Contraindicated in patients with hypersensitivity to other NSAIDs
- Alcohol may increase ulcerogenic effects if used concurrently
- May take 2 weeks or more to notice improvement
- Rx; Preg Cat C

• •

Side Effects

Headache	Blood dyscrasias	Rash
Nausea, anorexia	Hives	
GI bleeding	Facial swelling	

Nursing Considerations

- Treatment of rheumatoid arthritis, osteoarthritis, primary dysmenorrhea, gout, dental pain, musculoskeletal disorders, fever, headache, menstrual cramps
- Onset: 30 minutes, peak 1–2 hours
- Contact clinician if blurred vision, ringing or roaring in ears, which may indicate toxicity
- Contact clinician if changes in urinary pattern, increased weight, edema, increased pain in joints, fever, blood in urine, which may indicate kidney damage
- Full therapeutic effect may take up to 1 month
- Avoid use with ASA, NSAIDs, and alcohol, which may precipitate GI bleeding
- Take with food or milk
- Possible cross-allergy with aspirin
- OTC, Rx; Preg Cat C

NAPROXEN
(na-<u>prox</u>-en)

**(Aleve [OTC], Anaprox, Anaprox-DS,
EC-Naprosyn, Naprosyn)**

• •

METHOTREXATE
(meth-oh-<u>trex</u>-ate)

(Trexall)

Side Effects

GI bleeding

Blood dyscrasias

Hives

Rash

Asthma

Nursing Considerations

- Management of mild to moderate pain; treatment of rheumatoid, juvenile, and gouty arthritis, osteoarthritis, primary dysmenorrhea
- Patients with asthma, ASA hypersensitivity, or nasal polyps have increased risk of hypersensitivity
- Contact clinician if blurred vision, ringing or roaring in ears, which may indicate toxicity
- Contact clinician if black stools, flulike symptoms
- Contact clinician if changes in urinary pattern, increased weight, edema, increased pain in joints, fever, blood in urine, which may indicate kidney damage
- Use sunscreen to prevent photosensitivity
- Avoid use with ASA, steroids, and alcohol
- OTC, Rx; Preg Cat C

· ·

Side Effects

Nausea, vomiting, diarrhea

Anorexia

Alopecia

Ulcerative stomatitis

Dizziness

Nursing Considerations

- Treatment of cancer, mycosis fungoides, psoriasis, rheumatoid arthritis
- PO, IM, IV: onset 4–7 days, peak 7–14 days, duration 21 days
- Avoid crowds or people with known infections
- Do not take with ASA or other NSAIDs which may cause GI bleeding
- Monitor for pulmonary toxicity, which may manifest early as a dry, nonproductive cough
- Rx; Preg Cat X

TAMOXIFEN
(ta-<u>mox</u>-i-fen)

· ·

Cardiovascular Medications
ACE Inhibitors

BENAZEPRIL HCL
(ben-<u>as</u>-uh-pril)

(Lotensin)

Side Effects

Nausea, vomiting
Hot flashes
Rash
Vaginal discharge

Irregular menses
Fluid retention
Depression,
  mood disturbances

Nursing Considerations

- Management of advanced breast cancer not responsive to other therapy in estrogen-receptor-positive patients
- Peak 4–7 hours
- To decrease GI upset, take after antacid, after evening meal, before bedtime, or take antiemetic 30–60 minutes ahead
- Vaginal bleeding, pruritus, hot flashes are reversible after stopping med
- Contact clinician if decreased visual acuity, which may be irreversible
- Tumor flare (increase in tumor size and increased bone pain) may occur, but will decrease rapidly; may take analgesics for pain
- Rx; Preg Cat D

• •

Side Effects

Angioedema
Cough
Headache

Dizziness
Fatigue

Nursing Considerations

- Used to treat hypertension
- Often used in combination with thiazide diuretics
- Indomethacin may decrease therapeutic effects
- Avoid potassium containing salt substitutes because of potassium-sparing effect
- Avoid nonprescription cough medications unless physician directed
- Rx; Preg Cat D

CAPTOPRIL
(<u>kap</u>-toe-pril)

(Capoten)

• •

ENALAPRIL
(e-<u>nal</u>-a-pril)

(Vasotec)

Side Effects

Bronchospasm, dyspnea, cough
Orthostatic hypotension
Dizziness

Tachycardia
Loss of taste

Nursing Considerations

- Treatment of hypertension, CHF, left ventricular dysfunction after MI, diabetic neuropathy
- Contact clinician if fever, skin rash, sore throat, mouth sores, swelling of hands or feet, fast or irregular heartbeat, chest pain, or cough
- Take on empty stomach 1 hour before meals or 2 hours after; tablets may be crushed and mixed with juice or soft food for ease of swallowing
- Loss of taste might last for first 2–3 months, clinical concern is interference with nutrition
- Avoid changing positions (sitting/standing/lying) rapidly, esp. during the first few days before body adjusts to med
- Do not use OTC (cough, cold, or allergy) meds unless directed by clinician
- Avoid potassium supplements and potassium salt substitute
- Rx; Preg Cat First Trimester C; Preg Cat Second Trimester D

• •

Side Effects

Headache
Dizziness, hypotension
Tachycardia
Tinnitus

Hyperkalemia
Angioedema
Persistent cough

Nursing Considerations

- Treatment of hypertension, CHF, left ventricular dysfunction
- Contact clinician if fever, skin rash, sore throat, mouth sores, swelling of hands or feet, fast or irregular heartbeat, chest pain, or cough
- Avoid changing positions (sitting/standing/lying) rapidly, esp. during the first few days before body adjusts to med
- Cardiovascular adverse reactions may reoccur
- Do not use OTC (cough, cold, or allergy) meds unless directed by clinician
- Avoid potassium supplements and potassium salt substitutes
- Rx; Preg Cat First Trimester C; Preg Cat Second Trimester D

FOSINOPRIL
(foh-<u>sin</u>-oh-prill)

(Monopril)

· ·

LISINOPRIL
(lye-<u>sin</u>-oh-pril)

(Prinivil, Zestril)

Side Effects

Headache

Dizziness, fatigue

Nausea, vomiting, diarrhea

Angioedema

Hepatic failure

Cough

Nursing Considerations

- Treatment of hypertension, adjunct in treating CHF when not responding to usual meds
- Take at the same time each day; peaks at 2–6 hours
- Initial response might include dizziness and lightheadedness
- Avoid salt substitutes containing potassium
- Change positions (sitting/standing/lying) slowly
- Contact clinician if sore throat, swelling of hands and feet, chest pain, mouth sores, irregular heartbeat
- Rx; Preg Cat C First Trimester; Preg Cat D Second and Third Trimesters

• •

Side Effects

Headache

Dizziness

Nausea, vomiting, diarrhea

Hypotension

Tachycardia

Fatigue

SIADH

Cough

Nursing Considerations

- Treatment of mild to moderate hypertension, systolic CHF, acute MI
- Avoid changing positions (lying/sitting/standing) rapidly
- May take without regard to food
- Avoid high-sodium foods (canned soups, lunch meats, cheese)
- Avoid high-potassium foods (bananas, citrus fruits, raisins)
- Rx; Preg Cat First Trimester C; Preg Cat Second Trimester D

RAMIPRIL
(<u>ram</u>-ih-prill)

(Altace)

· ·

DOXAZOSIN MESYLATE
(dox-<u>ay</u>-zoe-sin)

(Cardura)

Side Effects

Headache   Nausea
Hypotension   Cough
Dizziness   Fatigue
Vertigo

Nursing Considerations

- Treatment of hypertension, CHF following MI, reduce risk of death from CV causes in patients with risk factors
- Can mix capsule contents with water, juice, or applesauce to aid swallowing
- Avoid changing positions (lying/sitting/standing) rapidly
- Contact clinician if persistent, dry, nonproductive cough; increased SOB; edema; or unusual bruising or bleeding
- Avoid salt substitutes containing potassium
- Rx; Preg Cat C First Trimester; Preg Cat D Second and Third Trimesters

• •

Side Effects

Dizziness   Fatigue, malaise
Headache   Priapism (rare)

Nursing Considerations

- Treatment of hypertension, benign prostatic hyperplasia (BPH)
- Avoid changing positions (lying/sitting/standing) rapidly
- Can have first-dose syncope, maintain recumbent for 90 minutes
- Full therapeutic effects may require several weeks of therapy
- Avoid high-sodium foods (canned soups, lunch meats, cheese)
- Use caution in potentially hazardous activities until stabilized
- Avoid alcohol, smoking
- Wear medical information tag
- Rx; Preg Cat C

PRAZOSIN HCL
(<u>pray</u>-zoh-sin)

(Minipress)

• •

TERAZOSIN HCL
(ter-<u>ay</u>-zoh-sin)

(Hytrin)

Side Effects

Dizziness

Nausea, vomiting, diarrhea

Drowsiness

Headache

Palpitations

Syncope

Nursing Considerations

- Treatment of hypertension
- Onset 2 hours, peak 1–3 hours, duration 6–12 hours
- Can have first-dose syncope, take the first dose (and any increment) at bedtime, do not drive for 24 hours
- Full therapeutic effects may require 4–6 weeks of therapy
- Food may delay absorption
- Avoid changing positions (lying/sitting/standing) rapidly
- Check with clinician before using OTC cold, cough, and allergy meds
- Rx; Preg Cat C

• •

Side Effects

Dizziness

Headache

Drowsiness

Nausea

Weakness

Syncope

Nursing Considerations

- Treatment of hypertension, BPH
- Avoid changing positions (lying/sitting/standing) rapidly
- Can have first-dose syncope, take the first dose (and any increment) at bedtime; do not drive or operate machinery for 4 hours
- Rx; Preg Cat C

VALSARTAN
(val-<u>sar</u>-tan)

(Diovan)

- -

VALSARTAN HYDROCHLOROTHIAZIDE
(val-<u>sar</u>-tan hahy-druh-klawr-uh-thahy-uh-zahyd)

(Diovan HCT)

Side Effects

Headache

Dizziness

Excessive tiredness;
fatigue

Stomach, back, or
joint pain

Nausea, vomiting,
diarrhea

Hypotension

Viral infection

Cough,
flu symptoms

High blood
creatinine

Rash

Vasculitis

Nursing Considerations

- Treatment of hypertension; heart failure for patients who cannot
  take an ACE inhibitor, reduction of cardiovascular mortality
  in patients with left ventricular failure, or left ventricular
  dysfunction after MI
- Take once daily for high blood pressure; twice daily for
  heart failure
- Avoid salt substitutes containing potassium
- Monitor blood creatine; may decrease kidney function
- May have cross-allergy to sulfonamides
- Rx; Preg Cat D

• •

Side Effects

Headache

Dizziness

Excessive tiredness;
fatigue

Stomach, back, or
joint pain

Nausea, vomiting,
diarrhea

Hypotension

Viral infection

Cough,
flu symptoms

High blood
creatinine

Rash

Blurred vision

Nasopharyngitis

Tinnitus, vertigo

GI distress

Male sexual
dysfunction

Nursing Considerations

- Treatment of hypertension; heart failure for patients who cannot
  take an ACE inhibitor
- Take once daily for high blood pressure; twice daily for heart failure
- Avoid salt substitutes containing potassium
- Monitor blood sugars in diabetic patients; may cause hyperglycemia
- NSAIDs may reduce the effect of diuretic
- May cause exacerbation of SLE
- May have cross-allergy to sulfonamides
- Rx; Preg Cat D

ISOSORBIDE DINITRATE
(eye-soe-<u>sor</u>-bide)

(Isordil)

· ·

ISOSORBIDE MONONITRATE
(eye-soe-<u>sor</u>-bide)

(Ismo)

Side Effects

Dizziness, postural hypotension   Nausea
Vascular headache, flushing   Lightheadedness
Drowsiness

Nursing Considerations

- Treatment/prophylaxis of angina pectoris, CHF
- PO: 1 hour before food or 2 hours after meals for maximum absorption, but taking with food may reduce or eliminate headache
- Chewable tablet: chew well, hold in mouth for 2 minutes before swallowing
- Sublingual: dissolve under tongue, do not eat, drink, talk or smoke during use, go to ED if pain not relieved in 15 minutes
- Avoid changing positions (lying/sitting/standing) rapidly
- Use caution in potentially hazardous activities until stabilized
- Avoid alcohol, smoking, strenuous exercise in hot environment
- Wear medical information tag
- Rx; Preg Cat C

• •

Side Effects

Dizziness, postural hypotension   Drowsiness
Vascular headache, flushing   Nausea

Nursing Considerations

- Treatment/prophylaxis of angina pectoris
- PO: 1 hour before food or 2 hours after meals for maximum absorption, but taking with food may reduce or eliminate headache
- Chewable tablet: chew well, hold in mouth for 2 minutes before swallowing
- Sublingual: dissolve under tongue; do not eat, drink, talk, or smoke during use; go to ED if pain not relieved in 15 minutes
- Avoid changing positions (lying/sitting/standing) rapidly
- Use caution in potentially hazardous activities until stabilized
- Avoid alcohol, smoking, strenuous exercise in hot environment
- Wear medical information tag
- Rx; Preg Cat C

NITROGLYCERIN
(nye-troe-<u>gli</u>-ser-in)

(Nitro-Par, Transderm-Nitro/Nitrostat)

• •

Cardiovascular Medications
Antiarrhythmics

AMIODARONE HCL
(am-ee-<u>oh</u>-da-rone)

(Cordarone, Pacerone)

Side Effects

Transient headache   Flushing
Postural hypotension

Nursing Considerations

- Treatment/prophylaxis of angina pectoris; IV used for control of BP during surgery and CHF associated with acute MI
- Sustained-release: take every 6 to 12 hours on an empty stomach; onset 20–45 minutes, duration 3–8 hours
- Sublingual: patient sitting/lying should let tablet dissolve under tongue and not swallow saliva; onset 1–3 minutes, duration 30 minutes
- Spray: hold canister vertically, spray on tongue, close mouth immediately, do not inhale spray; onset 2 minutes, duration 30–60 minutes
- IV: use infusion pump and special non-PVC tubing; onset 1–2 minutes, duration 3–5 minutes
- Ointment: spread on skin in thin uniform layer; onset 30–60 minutes, duration 2–12 hours
- Transdermal: apply to clean hairless area; rotate sites; onset 30–60 minutes, duration 12–24 hours
- Go to ED if pain not relieved with three tablets in 15 minutes
- Wear medical information tag
- Rx; Preg Cat C

• •

Side Effects

Dizziness, fatigue, malaise   Neurologic dysfunction
Corneal microdeposits   Muscle weakness
Bradycardia, hypotension   Cardiac arrest
Anorexia, constipation   Nausea, vomiting
Photosensitivity

Nursing Considerations

- Management of ventricular arrhythmias unresponsive to less toxic agents
- IV: continuous cardiac monitoring
- Assess for signs of pulmonary toxicity: rales/crackles, decreased breath sounds, pleuritic friction rub, fatigue, dyspnea, cough, pleuritic pain, fever
- Neurotoxicity (ataxia, muscle weakness, tingling or numbness in fingers or toes, uncontrolled movements, tremors) common during initial therapy
- Side effects may not appear until several days, weeks, or years and may persist for several months after stopping med
- Teach patient to check radial pulse
- Use sunscreen and protective clothing to prevent photosensitivity
- May increase ALT, AST
- Rx; Preg Cat D

LIDOCAINE HCL
(<u>lye</u>-doe-kane)

(Xylocaine)

. . . .

PROCAINAMIDE
(proe-<u>kane</u>-a-mide)

Side Effects

Hypotension, tremors
Double vision
Tinnitus
Respiratory depression/arrest
Confusion, blurred vision

Drowsiness, dizziness
Twitching, convulsions
Bradycardia
Visual color disturbances

Nursing Considerations

- Used for premature ventricular contractions
- Give oxygen; have resuscitation equipment available
- IV: use infusion pump; patient on cardiac monitor
- Check BUN, creatinine
- Monitor lungs for rales
- Rx; Preg Cat B

• •

Side Effects

Hypotension
Bradycardia
Nausea, vomiting

Fever, rash
Dizziness
Neutropenia

Anxiety

Nursing Considerations

- Management of life-threatening ventricular dysrhythmias and maintain NSR following conversion of atrial arrhythmia
- IV: use infusion pump; monitor BP every 5 to 15 minutes; on cardiac monitor; keep patient recumbent
- IV: monitor CBC, blood levels, I & O, daily weight
- PO: best absorption on empty stomach, may take with food to decrease GI upset
- Take at equal intervals around the clock
- Teach patient to check radial pulse
- Avoid caffeine
- May increase alkaline phosphatase, bilirium, lactic dehydrogenase, AST
- Rx; Preg Cat C

QUINIDINE
(<u>kwin</u>-i-deen)

• •

Cardiovascular Medications
Antiarrhythmics

SOTALOL
(<u>soe</u>-ta-lole)

(Betapace)

Side Effects

Anemia

Hypotension

Nausea, vomiting, diarrhea

Headache

Heart block

Tinnitus

Fever

Fatigue

Vision changes

Nursing Considerations

- Used for atrial or ventricular arrhythmias and to test malaria
- May increase toxicity for digitalis
- Monitor liver function tests and I & 0
- Check apical pulse and BP
- Monitor EKG and BP
- Avoid changing positions (lying/sitting/standing) rapidly
- Avoid use with alcohol, caffeine, smoking
- Patient should wear medical information tag
- Rx; Preg Cat C

• •

Side Effects

Fatigue

Weakness

Impotence

Bradycardia

Dyspnea

Life-threatening ventricular arrhythmias

Hyperglycemia

Nursing Considerations

- Management of life-threatening ventricular arrhythmias
- Teach patient to check radial pulse; if less than 50, hold med and contact clinician
- Change positions (sitting/standing/lying) slowly
- Avoid activities that require alertness until drug response known
- Contact clinician if slow pulse, difficulty breathing, wheezing, cold hands and feet, dizziness, confusion, depression, rash, fever, sore throat, unusual bleeding or bruising
- Milk products may decrease absorption
- Rx; Preg Cat B

BISOPROLOL
(bis-<u>oh</u>-pro-lole)

(Zebeta)

• •

CLONIDINE PATCH
(<u>kloe</u>-ni-deen)

**(Catapres; also available
as Catapres TTS oral tablets)**

Side Effects

GI upset   Dizziness
Fatigue   Headache
Weakness

Nursing Considerations

- Treatment of mild to moderate hypertension
- Peak: 2–4 hours
- Therapeutic response in 1 to 2 weeks
- Do not stop med abruptly; may precipitate angina
- Do not use OTC meds with stimulants, such as nasal decongestants, OTC cold meds, unless directed
- Avoid alcohol, smoking, sodium intake
- Contact clinician if signs of CHF: difficulty breathing, night cough, swelling of extremities
- Rx; Preg Cat C

• •

Side Effects

Drowsiness, sedation   Dizziness
Severe rebound hypertension   Headache
Dry mouth and eyes   Constipation

Nursing Considerations

- Treatment of hypertension, severe cancer pain (in combination with opiates)
- Avoid changing positions (lying/sitting/standing) rapidly
- Avoid use with alcohol, CNS depressants
- Avoid high-sodium foods (canned soups, lunch meats, cheese)
- Use caution in potentially hazardous activities
- Avoid alcohol, smoking, strenuous exercise in hot environment
- Apply patch to nonhairy area (upper outer arm, anterior chest), rotate sites, do not apply to scarred or irritated area
- Wear medical information tag
- Caution patients who wear contact lens that drug may cause dry eyes
- May cause a positive Coombs test
- Rx; Preg Cat C

HYDRALAZINE HCL
(hye-<u>dral</u>-a-zeen)

HYDROCHLOROTHIAZIDE/ LISINOPRIL
(hye-droe-klor-oh-<u>thye</u>-a-zide/
lye-<u>sin</u>-oh-pril)

(Prinzide, Zestoretic)

Side Effects

Headache
Palpitations, tachycardia, angina
Edema
Lupus erythematosus-like
  syndrome
Anorexia

Tremors
Dizziness
Anxiety
Flushing
Rash
Nausea, vomiting, diarrhea

Nursing Considerations

- Used to treat essential hypertension; also for heart valve replacement and treatment of CHF
- PO: give with meals to enhance absorption
- Observe mental status
- Check for weight gain, edema
- Avoid changing positions (lying/sitting/standing) rapidly
- Contact clinician if chest pain, severe fatigue, fever, muscle, or joint pain
- Do not confuse with hydroxyzine
- Rx; Preg Cat C

• •

Side Effects

Headache
Dizziness
Nausea, vomiting, diarrhea
Hypotension
Tachycardia

Fatigue
Cough
Muscle cramps
Angioedema

Nursing Considerations

- Used to treat essential hypertension
- Avoid changing positions (lying/sitting/standing) rapidly
- May take without regard to food
- Avoid high-sodium foods (canned soups, lunch meats, cheese)
- Avoid high-potassium foods (bananas, citrus fruits, raisins)
- Rx; Preg Cat C First Trimester; Preg Cat D Second and Third Trimesters

MINOXIDIL
(mi-<u>nox</u>-i-dill)

(as topical, Rogaine)

• •

ATORVASTATIN CALCIUM
(a-<u>tore</u>-vuh-stat-in)

(Lipitor)

Side Effects

Edema

Rash

Increase in body hair

Nursing Considerations

- Teach patient to take radial pulse
- Check for weight gain, edema
- Topical application (Rogaine) approved to promote hair growth in men and women
- Do not use on children or infants
- Avoid contact with eyes, mucous membranes, or sensitive skin areas
- OTC, Rx; Preg Cat C

. . . .

Side Effects

Constipation

Arthralgia

Decreased vitamins A, D, K

Myopathy

Abdominal pain

Nasopharyngitis

Nausea

UTI

Nursing Considerations

- Used to lower cholesterol levels, digitalis toxicity, biliary obstruction pruritus, and diarrhea; decrease risk of MI and stroke in patient with diabetes type 2
- Take other meds 1 hour before or 4 hours after this med to avoid poor absorption
- Mix granules in applesauce or liquid, do not take dry, let stand for 2 minutes
- Monitor for hypoprothrombinemia: bleeding gums, tarry stools, hematuria, bruising
- Monitor liver enzymes
- Avoid grapefruit products
- Rx; Preg Cat X

COLESTIPOL
(koe-<u>les</u>-ti-pole)

(Colestid)

• •

FENOFIBRATE
(fen-oh-<u>fye</u>-brate)

(TriCor, Fenoglide, Lipofen, Triglide)

Side Effects

Constipation

Decreased vitamins A, D, K

Pruritus

Abdominal pain

Nausea

Diarrhea

Nursing Considerations

- Used to lower cholesterol levels, digitalis toxicity, biliary obstruction
- Take other meds 1 hour before or 4 hours after this med to avoid poor absorption
- Mix granules in applesauce or liquid, do not take dry, let stand for 2 minutes
- Monitor for hypoprothrombinemia: bleeding gums, tarry stools, hematuria, bruising
- Do not crush, cut, or chew tablets; drink plenty of liquid
- Rx; Preg Cat N/A

· ·

Side Effects

Nausea, vomiting, diarrhea, constipation

Headache

Heartburn

Pain in the back, arms, or legs

Nursing Considerations

- Used to lower total cholesterol, triglycerides, LDL cholesterol; used to increase HDL cholesterol
- Take once daily, with or without food
- May stop if no improvement in 2 months
- Used in conjunction with low cholesterol and low saturated fat diet regimen
- Teach patient to report unexplained muscle pain
- Monitor prothrombin levels in warfarin therapy
- Monitor liver function tests
- Rx; Preg Cat C

GEMFIBROZIL
(jem-fi-broe-zil)

(Lopid)

· ·

LOVASTATIN
(loh-vah-stat-in)

(Mevacor)

Side Effects

Abdominal pain, diarrhea
GI upset
Fatigue

Cholelithiasis
Nausea

Nursing Considerations

- Used to lower cholesterol levels; type IV and V hyperlipidemia
- Take 30 minutes before meals
- Check CBC and liver function tests
- PO: take 30 minutes before morning and evening meals
- May stop if no improvement in 3 months
- Rx; Preg Cat C

• •

Side Effects

Flatus, constipation
Abdominal pain, nausea,
    diarrhea, GI upset
Heartburn
Muscle cramps

Dizziness
Headache
Tremor
Blurred vision
Rash, pruritus

Nursing Considerations

- Used to lower cholesterol levels, primary and secondary prevention of coronary events
- Use sunscreen to prevent photosensitivity reactions
- Schedule liver function tests every 1 to 2 months during the first 1.5 years
- Onset 2 weeks, peak 4–6 weeks, duration 6 weeks
- Take with food, absorption is reduced by 30% on an empty stomach
- Contact clinician if unexplained muscle pain, tenderness or weakness, especially if with fever or malaise
- Rx; Preg Cat X

NIACIN
(<u>nye</u>-a-sin)

**(Niacor for immediate-release;
Niaspan for sustained-release)**

• •

NICOTINIC ACID
(nih-koh-<u>tin</u>-ick)

(Slo-Niacin, vitamin B)

Side Effects

Headache   Flushing
Nausea   Cough
Postural hypotension   Pruritus
Myopathy

Nursing Considerations

- Treatment of pellagra, hyperlipidemias, peripheral vascular disease
- Take with meals to reduce GI upset, can add 325 mg ASA 30 minutes before dose to reduce flushing
- Flushing will occur several hours after med taken, will decrease over 2 weeks
- Avoid changing positions (sitting/standing/lying) rapidly
- May be used in combination with simvastatin or lovastatin
- Monitor liver enzymes
- May increase glucose level
- OTC, Rx; Preg Cat C

• •

Side Effects

Headache   Flushing
Nausea   Dry skin
Postural hypotension

Nursing Considerations

- Treatment of pellagra, hyperlipidemias, peripheral vascular disease
- Take with meals to reduce GI upset, can add 325 mg ASA 30 minutes before dose to reduce flushing
- Flushing will occur several hours after med taken, will decrease over 2 weeks
- Avoid changing positions (sitting/standing/lying) rapidly
- Taking NSAIDs may reduce flushing
- May alter blood sugar
- Monitor liver enzymes
- OTC, Rx; Preg Cat C

PRAVASTATIN
(<u>pra</u>-va-sta-tin)

(Pravachol)

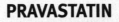

ROSUVASTATIN CALCIUM
(roe-sue-vuh-<u>stat</u>-in)

(Crestor)

Side Effects

Abdominal cramps, flatus   Constipation, diarrhea
Heartburn

Nursing Considerations

- Treatment of hypercholesterolemia, apolipoprotein B (apo B), risk reduction of recurrent MI, atherosclerosis
- Schedule liver function tests semiannually
- Take without regard to food
- Contact clinician if unexplained muscle pain, tenderness or weakness, especially if with fever or malaise
- Rx; Preg Cat X

. . . .

Side Effects

Myalgia   Nausea
Constipation   Myopathy
Abdominal pain   Rhabdomyolysis

Nursing Considerations

- Used as adjunct therapy to diet to reduce LDL cholesterol and increase HDL cholesterol; slow progression of atherosclerosis
- Patients should discontinue therapy and notify physician in case of pregnancy
- Use with caution in patients with a history of large alcohol consumption
- Liver function tests are recommended every 12 weeks
- Patient should keep tight control of diet during therapy
- May be used in children 10–17 years of age
- Asian patients may require lower dose to begin therapy
- Do not use with niacin
- Rx; Preg Cat X

SIMVASTATIN
(<u>sim</u>-va-sta-tin)

(Zocor)

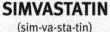

ATENOLOL
(a-<u>ten</u>-oh-lole)

(Tenormin, Tenoretic in combination with chlorthalidone)

Side Effects

Eye lens opacities
Liver dysfunction
URI
Headache

Abdominal pain
Constipation
Nausea

Nursing Considerations

- Treatment of hypercholesterolemia, hypertriglyceridemia, hyperlipoproteinemias, coronary artery disease
- Have eye exam before, 1 month after, and then annually after starting med
- Schedule liver function tests semiannually
- Take without regard to food
- Contact clinician if unexplained muscle pain, tenderness or weakness, especially with fever or malaise
- Asian patients should not take niacin while taking simvastatin
- Rx; Preg Cat X

• •

Side Effects

Bradycardia, cold extremities
Postural hypotension
Bronchospasm in overdose
2nd- or 3rd-degree heart block
Cold extremities

Insomnia, fatigue
Dizziness
Mental changes
Nausea, diarrhea
CHF

Nursing Considerations

- Used in treatment of hypertension, MI, prophylaxis of angina
- Masks signs of hypoglycemia in diabetics
- Teach patient how to take radial pulse
- Check pulse, if less than 50 beats per minute, hold the med and contact clinician
- PO: take before meals, at bedtime
- Tablet may be crushed or swallowed whole
- Do not stop abruptly; taper over 2 weeks
- Rx; Preg Cat D

CARVEDILOL
(kar-<u>ved</u>-i-lole)

(Coreg)

• •

METOPROLOL SUCCINATE
(meh-<u>toe</u>-proe-lole)

(Toprol XL, the sustained-release form)

Side Effects

Dizziness	Fatigue
Diarrhea	CHF worsening
Postural hypotension	Dry eyes
Impotence	Bradycardia
Hyperglycemia	

Nursing Considerations

- Used in treatment of hypertension, CHF, LV dysfunction after MI
- PO: take with food
- Tablet may be crushed or swallowed whole
- Do not stop abruptly; taper over 1 to 2 weeks
- May mask symptoms of low blood sugar in diabetes
- May mask symptoms of hyperthyroidism
- Rx; Preg Cat C

• •

Side Effects

Bradycardia, palpitations	Depression
Nausea, vomiting, diarrhea	Insomnia
Hypotension	Dizziness
CHF	Confusion

Nursing Considerations

- Used in treatment of hypertension, MI (IV use), prophylaxis of angina, heart failure
- Teach patient how to take radial pulse
- Check pulse, if less than 50 beats per minute, hold the med and contact clinician
- PO: may be taken with food
- Tablet must be swallowed whole
- Do not stop abruptly; taper over 2 weeks; may precipitate angina
- Do not use OTC products (nasal decongestants, cold preparations) unless directed by prescriber
- May worsen heart failure
- May worsen hypoglycemia in diabetes
- Report any dyspnea
- Rx; Preg Cat C

METOPROLOL TARTRATE
(meh-<u>toe</u>-proe-lole)

(Lopressor, the immediate-release form)

. . . .

PROPRANOLOL HCL
(proe-<u>pran</u>-oh-lole)

(Inderal)

Side Effects

Bradycardia, palpitations	Nausea, vomiting, diarrhea	Dizziness
Hypotension	Depression	Constipation
CHF	Insomnia	

Nursing Considerations

- Used in treatment of hypertension, MI (IV use), prophylaxis of angina
- Teach patient how to take radial pulse
- Check pulse, if less than 50 beats per minute, hold the med and contact clinician
- PO: take on an empty stomach, before meals, at bedtime
- Tablet may be crushed or swallowed whole
- Do not stop abruptly; taper over 2 weeks; may precipitate angina
- Do not use OTC products (nasal decongestants, cold preparations) unless directed by prescriber
- May mask hypoglycemia in diabetics
- Report any dyspnea
- Rx; Preg Cat C

• •

Side Effects

Weakness	Bronchospasm	Depression
Hypotension	Bradycardia	

Nursing Considerations

- Used in treatment of stable angina, hypertension, dysrhythmias, migraine, prophylaxis MI, essential tremor, alcohol withdrawal, atrial fibrillation
- Teach patient how to take radial pulse
- Check pulse, if less than 50 beats per minute, hold the med and contact clinician
- PO: take with full glass of water at the same time each day
- Do not open, chew, crush extended-release capsule
- Do not stop abruptly; taper over 2 weeks; may precipitate life-threatening dysrhythmias
- Do not use aluminum-containing antacid; may decrease absorption
- May cause cardiac failure
- May cause hypoglycemia in diabetics
- May mask hyperthyroidism
- Rx; Preg Cat C

SOTALOL
(<u>soe</u>-ta-lole)
(Betapace)

• •

Cardiovascular Medications
Calcium Channel Blockers

AMLODIPINE BESYLATE
(am-<u>loh</u>-dip-ene)
(Norvasc)

Side Effects

Fatigue
Weakness
Impotence
Bradycardia

Dyspnea
Life-threatening, ventricular
 arrhythmias
Hyperglycemia

Nursing Considerations

- Management of life-threatening ventricular arrhythmias
- Teach patient to check radial pulse
- Check pulse; if less than 50 beats per minute, hold med and contact clinician
- Change positions (sitting/standing/lying) slowly
- Avoid activities that require alertness until drug response known
- Contact clinician if slow pulse, difficulty breathing, wheezing, cold hands and feet, dizziness, confusion, depression, rash, fever, sore throat, unusual bleeding or bruising
- Milk products may decrease absorption
- Rx; Preg Cat B

• •

Side Effects

Flushing
Edema
Headache
Fatigue

Nausea, vomiting
Abdominal pain
Somnolence

Nursing Considerations

- Used to treat hypertension and documented CAD
- Used also to treat vasospastic angina pectoris
- May be taken without regard to meal
- Consult physician before taking nonprescription cough remedies
- Do not store in bathroom
- Rx; Preg Cat C

DILTIAZEM HCL
(dil-<u>tye</u>-a-zem)

**(Cardizem, Dilacor, Tiazac,
Cardizem CD [once a day])**

• •

FELODIPINE
(fe-<u>loe</u>-di-peen)

Side Effects

Hypotension, dizziness

Edema

Nausea, constipation

Rash

Headache

Fatigue, drowsiness

Angioedema

Bradycardia

Nursing Considerations

- Management of angina, hypertension, vasospasm, atrial fibrillation, flutter, paroxysmal supraventricular tachycardia
- Reduces workload of left ventricle, coronary vasodilator
- Monitor blood pressure during dosage adjustments
- PO: take on an empty stomach, with a full glass of water
- Teach patient how to take radial pulse and keep records of pulse rate
- Avoid hazardous activities until stabilized on drug
- Do not crush, chew, or break
- May increase ALT, AST, LDH, CPK, and alkaline phosphatase
- Rx; Preg Cat C

• •

Side Effects

Dysrhythmia

Headache

Fatigue

Edema

Flushing

Nursing Considerations

- Used in treatment of essential hypertension, angina
- Do not adjust dosage at intervals of less than 2 weeks
- PO: take without regard to meals
- Do not open, chew, or crush extended-release capsule
- Do not use OTC products or alcohol unless directed by prescriber; limit caffeine
- May increase ALT
- Rx; Preg Cat C

NIFEDIPINE

(nye-<u>fed</u>-i-peen)

(Adalat CC, Procardia XL)

• •

Cardiovascular Medications
Calcium Channel Blockers

VERAPAMIL HCL

(ver-<u>ap</u>-a-mill)

(Calan, Covera)

Side Effects

Orthostatic hypotension	Chest pain	Nausea
Peripheral edema	Headache, dizziness	Rash
Leg cramps	Impotence	
	Fatigue	

Nursing Considerations

- Used in treatment of hypertension, angina
- Avoid changing positions (sitting/standing/lying) rapidly
- PO: take on an empty stomach; onset 20 minutes, peak 30 minutes to 6 hours, duration 6–8 hours
- PO of extended-release capsule: do not open, chew, crush; can take without regard to meals; duration of 24 hours; shell may appear in stools, but is insignificant
- Do not use OTC products or alcohol unless directed by prescriber; limit caffeine
- Monitor BP when used with beta blockers
- May cause CHF when used with beta blockers
- Do not drink grapefruit juice; stop grapefruit juice at least 3 days prior to initiating nifedipine therapy
- Do not take with St. John's wort
- Rx; Preg Cat C

• •

Side Effects

Edema	Drowsiness	Dizziness
Nausea, constipation	Fatigue	
Headache	URI	

Nursing Considerations

- Management of hypertension and angina
- PO: take before meals, except sustained-release which is to be taken with food
- Do not open, chew, or crush sustained- or extended-release capsule
- Teach patient how to take radial pulse and keep records of pulse rate
- Avoid hazardous activities until stabilized on drug
- Do not use OTC products or alcohol unless directed by prescriber; limit caffeine
- Rx; Preg Cat C

DIGOXIN
(di-<u>jox</u>-in)

(Lanoxin)

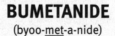

Cardiovascular Medications
Loop Diuretics

BUMETANIDE
(byoo-<u>met</u>-a-nide)

Side Effects

Headache	Nausea	Mental disturbances
Hypotension	Atrial tachycardia	Vomiting
Fatigue	(in children)	
Bradycardia	Dizziness	

Nursing Considerations

- Used in treatment of CHF, atrial fibrillation, flutter, or tachycardia
- Check pulse, if less than 60 beats per minute (adult) or 90 beats per minute (infant), hold the med and contact clinician
- PO: with or without food; may crush tablets and mix with food/fluids
- Do not open, chew, or crush capsule
- Contact clinician if loss of appetite, lower stomach pain, diarrhea, weakness, drowsiness, headache, blurred or yellow vision, rash, depression
- Eat a sodium-restricted and potassium-rich (bananas, orange juice) diet to keep potassium level normal
- Avoid OTC meds and herbal meds; many adverse interactions may occur
- Rx; Preg Cat C

• •

Side Effects

Potassium depletion	Ototoxicity	Hives
Electrolyte imbalance	Hyperglycemia	Muscle weakness
Hypovolemia	Hypotension	Tinnitus

Nursing Considerations

- Treatment of edema, adult nocturia
- PO: diuresis onset 30–60 minutes, peak 1–2 hours, duration 3–6 hours
- IM: diuresis onset 40 minutes, peak 1–2 hours, duration 4–6 hours
- IV: diuresis onset 5 minutes, peak 15–30 minutes, duration 3–6 hours
- Weigh daily
- Do not take at bedtime to prevent nocturia
- Encourage potassium-containing foods
- May increase LDL, cholesterol, and triglycerides
- May increase HDL
- Monitor BUN, CBC, calcium, and uric acid
- Monitor for hearing loss
- Rx; Preg Cat C

FUROSEMIDE
(fur-<u>oh</u>-se-mide)

(Lasix)

. . . .

CLOPIDOGREL
(klo-<u>pid</u>-oh-grel)

(Plavix)

Side Effects

Hypotension
Hypokalemia
Hyperglycemia
Nausea

Polyuria
Rash, pruritus
Muscle spasm

Nursing Considerations

- Used in treatment of pulmonary edema and edema in other conditions; hypertension
- PO: diuresis onset 60 minutes, peak 1–2 hours, duration 6–8 hours
- IV: diuresis onset 5 minutes, peak 30 minutes, duration 2 hours
- PO: take with food or milk to prevent GI upset, slightly lessened absorption, tablets may be crushed
- Take early in the day to prevent nocturia and sleeplessness
- Avoid changing positions (sitting/standing/lying) rapidly
- Use sunscreen or protective clothing to prevent photosensitivity
- NSAIDs may decrease effects
- Monitor blood sugar in diabetics
- Do not give IV faster than 4 mg/min; may cause ototoxicity
- Rx; Preg Cat C

• •

Side Effects

GI bleeding
Nausea, vomiting, diarrhea, GI discomfort
Depression

Bleeding, including life-threatening bleeding
Rash

Nursing Considerations

- Used to reduce risk of stroke, MI, peripheral artery disease in high risk patients, ACS
- Monitor blood studies in long-term therapy
- Take with meals or just after to decrease gastric symptoms
- Report signs of unusual bruising, bleeding; it may take longer to stop bleeding
- Rx; Preg Cat B

DIPYRIDAMOLE
(dye-peer-<u>id</u>-a-mole)

(Persantine)

• •

TICLOPIDINE HCL
(ty-<u>cloe</u>-pi-deen)

Side Effects

Headache	Nausea, vomiting
Dizziness	Postural hypotension
Weakness, fainting, syncope	Rash

Nursing Considerations

- Prevention of transient ischemic attacks, MIs, with warfarin in heart valves, with ASA in bypass grafts
- PO: peak in 2 to 2.5 hours; duration 6 hours
- PO: on an empty stomach, 1 hour before or 2 hours after meals with full glass of water
- Full therapeutic response may take several months
- IV: do not give more than 60 mg over 4 minutes
- Use caution with hazardous activities until stabilized on med
- Avoid changing positions (sitting/standing/lying) rapidly
- Intravenous aminophylline should be readily available to reverse effects of dipyridamole
- Rx; Preg Cat B

• •

Side Effects

Rash	Nausea
Diarrhea	Dyspnea
Bleeding	GI distress
Decrease in WBCs	Purpura
Thrombocytopenia	

Nursing Considerations

- Prevention of stroke in high-risk patients
- Monitor blood studies in long-term therapy
- Take with meals or just after to decrease gastric symptoms
- Monitor for signs of cholestasis (jaundice, dark urine, light-colored stools)
- May increase cholesterol and triglyceride levels
- Antacids may decrease effectiveness
- Rx; Preg Cat B

HYDROCHLOROTHIAZIDE/ TRIAMTERENE
(hye-droe-klor-oh-<u>thye</u>-a-zide/
trye-<u>am</u>-ter-een)

(Dyazide, Maxzide)

• •

Cardiovascular Medications
Potassium-Sparing/Combination Diuretics

SPIRONOLACTONE
(speer-in-oh-<u>lak</u>-tone)

(Aldactone)

Side Effects

Nausea, vomiting, diarrhea
Anemia
Renal stones
Hyperkalemia

Hyperglycemia
Glycosuria
Muscle cramps

Nursing Considerations

- Used in treatment of edema and hypertension
- Diuresis onset 2 hours
- Take with meals or just after to decrease gastric symptoms
- Take early in the day to prevent nocturia and sleeplessness
- Diabetes mellitus may become manifest during thiazide treatment
- May increase BUN and serum creatinine
- Rx; Preg Cat C

• •

Side Effects

Hyperkalemia
Hyponatremia
Vomiting, diarrhea

Bleeding
Rash, pruritus
Gynecomastia

Nursing Considerations

- Used in treatment of edema and hypertension, primary hyperaldosteronism
- Diuresis onset 24–48 hours, peak 48–72 hours
- Take in the morning to avoid interference with sleep
- Take with meals or just after to decrease gastric symptoms
- Avoid food high in potassium: oranges, bananas, salt substitutes, dried apricots, dates
- Weigh daily to determine fluid loss; effect of drug may be decreased if used daily
- Contact clinician if cramps, lethargy, menstrual abnormalities, deepening voice, breast enlargement
- Avoid potassium supplements
- Monitor electrolytes
- Rx; Preg Cat C

CHLORTHALIDONE
(klor-<u>thal</u>-i-done)

(Thalitone; Tenoretic in combination with atenolol)

. . . .

HYDROCHLOROTHIAZIDE
(hye-droe-klor-oh-<u>thye</u>-a-zide)

(Microzide)

Side Effects

Dizziness
Aplastic anemia
Orthostatic hypotension
Nausea, vomiting, anorexia

Urinary frequency
Fatigue, weakness
Electrolyte changes

Nursing Considerations

- Used in treatment of edema and hypertension
- Diuresis onset 2 hours, peak 6 hours, duration 24–72 hours
- Take with meals or just after to decrease gastric symptoms
- Blood sugar may increase in diabetics
- Take in the morning to avoid interference with sleep
- Weigh daily to determine fluid loss; effect of drug may be decreased if used daily
- May decrease PBI level
- Avoid changing positions (sitting/standing/lying) rapidly
- Rx; Preg Cat B

• •

Side Effects

Hypokalemia
Hyperglycemia
Nausea, vomiting, anorexia

Blurred vision
Fatigue, weakness
Confusion, esp. in elderly

Nursing Considerations

- Used in treatment of edema and hypertension
- Diuresis onset 2 hours, peak 4 hours, duration 6–12 hours
- Take with meals or just after to decrease gastric symptoms
- Blood sugar may increase in diabetics
- Take in morning to avoid interference with sleep
- Use sunscreen to prevent photosensitivity
- Monitor for signs of hypokalemia: postural hypotension, malaise, fatigue, tachycardia, leg cramps, weakness, dehydration
- Rx; Preg Cat B

INDAPAMIDE
(in-<u>dap</u>-a-mide)

. . . .

METOLAZONE
(me-<u>tole</u>-a-zone)

(Zaroxolyn—extended-release product)

Side Effects

Headache
Electrolyte changes
Orthostatic hypotension
Back pain
Gout
Muscle cramps

Cough
Rhinitis
Vision disturbances
Nausea
Rash, pruritus

Nursing Considerations

- Used in treatment of edema of CHF and hypertension
- Diuresis onset 1–2 hours, peak 2 hours, duration 36 hours
- Take with meals or just after to decrease gastric symptoms, slightly decreased absorption
- Avoid changing positions (sitting/standing/lying) rapidly
- Take in morning to avoid interference with sleep
- Monitor for signs of hypokalemia: postural hypotension, malaise, fatigue, tachycardia, leg cramps, weakness, dehydration
- Monitor electrolytes
- May cause hyperglycemia in diabetics
- Rx; Preg Cat B

• •

Side Effects

Dizziness, weakness, fatigue
Nausea, vomiting, anorexia
Rash

Hyperglycemia
Hypokalemia

Nursing Considerations

- Used in treatment of edema of CHF and hypertension, edema of renal diseases
- Diuresis onset 1 hour, peak 2 hours, duration 12–24 hours
- Take with meals or just after to decrease gastric symptoms, slightly decreased absorption
- Avoid changing positions (sitting/standing/lying) rapidly
- Take in morning to avoid interference with sleep
- Use sunscreen to prevent photosensitivity
- Monitor for signs of hypokalemia: postural hypotension, malaise, fatigue, tachycardia, leg cramps, weakness, dehydration
- May cause hyperglycemia in diabetics and latent diabetes
- Rx; Preg Cat B

ISOTRETINOIN
(eye-sew-<u>tret</u>-i-noyn)

(Claravis)

• •

KETOCONAZOLE
(key-toe-<u>koe</u>-na-zol)

(Nizoral)

Side Effects

Chilitis

Conjunctivitis

Dry skin

Dry mouth

Hair thinning

Cataracts

Aggression

Depression

Rash

Abnormal menses

Nursing Considerations

- Used to treat severe recalcitrant cystic acne that does not respond to conventional therapy, psoriasis, rosacea, basal cell carcinoma
- Women of child-bearing age must have a negative pregnancy test for each month of treatment
- Monitor for depression or suicidal thoughts
- Do not take vitamin A, may increase toxic effects
- May increase HDL, RBC, and WBC
- May increase FBs, platelets, ALT, AST
- Avoid St. John's wort
- Rx; Preg Cat X

• •

Side Effects

Dizziness

Photophobia

Rash

Nursing Considerations

- Treatment of fungal infections
- C & S before first dose
- PO: take early A.M. with food
- Also available as a topical cream or shampoo
- Cannot take within 2 hours of alkaline substances, requires acid media to dissolve, follow with glass of water
- Take at the same time each day
- To prevent photophobia in bright sunlight, wear sunglasses
- May require several weeks or months of therapy
- Avoid alcohol
- Do not allow shampoo to get in eyes
- Rx; Preg Cat C

NYSTATIN
(nye-<u>stat</u>-in)

(Mycostatin)

• •

FLUOCINONIDE
(floo-oh-<u>sin</u>-oh-nide)

(Lidex)

Side Effects

GI distress, hypersensitivity
Irritation (with topical use)

Nursing Considerations

- Treatment of *Candida* infections
- Discontinue if redness, swelling, irritation occurs
- Encourage good oral, vaginal, skin hygiene
- Do not mix oral suspension with food
- Rx; Preg Cat C (oral); Preg Cat A (vaginal)

• •

Side Effects

Acne   Striae
Atrophy   Burning
Epidermal thinning   Allergic dermatitis
Purpura

Nursing Considerations

- Topical glucocorticoid used to treat severe dermatoses not responding to less potent meds: psoriasis, eczema, contact dermatitis, pruritus
- Apply only to affected areas; do not get in eyes
- Leave site uncovered or lightly covered
- Occlusive dressing is not recommended, systemic absorption may occur
- Do not use on weeping, denuded, or infected areas
- Avoid sunlight on affected area
- Rx; Preg Cat C

TRIAMCINOLONE ACETONIDE
(trye-am-<u>sin</u>-oh-lone)

(Kenalog)

• •

ACARBOSE
(ay-<u>car</u>-bose)

(Precose)

Side Effects

Acne
Atrophy
Epidermal thinning
Purpura

Striae
Allergic contact dermatitis
Hypopigmentation

Nursing Considerations

- Topical glucocorticoid used to treat severe dermatoses not responding to less potent meds: psoriasis, eczema, contact dermatitis, pruritus
- Apply only to affected areas; do not get in eyes
- Leave site uncovered or lightly covered
- Occlusive dressing is not recommended, systemic absorption may occur
- Do not use on weeping, denuded, or infected areas
- Avoid sunlight on affected area
- Rx; Preg Cat C

• •

Side Effects

Abdominal pain
Diarrhea

Flatulence
Rash

Nursing Considerations

- Management of diabetes by non–insulin-dependent diabetics
- Used alone or in combination with a sulfonylurea or insulin
- PO: take with first bite of each meal, med blood level peaks in 1 hour
- Recognize signs of hypoglycemia: weakness, hunger, dizziness, tremors, anxiety, tachycardia, hunger, sweating
- Treat hypoglycemia with dextrose, or if severe, IV glucose or glucagon
- Measure short-term effectiveness with blood sugar 1 hour after meals
- Measure long-term effectiveness with glycosylated Hgb every 3 months for the first year
- Wear medical information tag
- Rx; Preg Cat B

GLIMEPIRIDE
(glye-<u>me</u>-pi-ride)

(Amaryl)

• •

GLIPIZIDE
(<u>glip</u>-i-zide)

(Glucotrol)

Side Effects

Headache
Weakness, dizziness
Drowsiness

Dyspnea
Fall in blood pressure
Shock

Nursing Considerations

- Management of stable type 2 diabetes mellitus
- Do not drink alcohol since it may produce a disulfiram reaction: nausea, headache, cramps, flushing, hypoglycemia
- Assess for symptoms of cholestatic jaundice: dark urine, pruritus, yellow sclera (rare)
- Take at breakfast or first main meal; onset is in 1 to 1.5 hours, peak in 1 to 3 hours, duration 10–24 hours
- Have a quick source of sugar or a glucagon emergency kit available
- Use sunscreen or protective clothing to prevent photosensitivity
- Do not crush, chew, or break extended-release tablet; its coating may appear in stool
- Cross-allergy possible if allergic to sulfonamide
- Monitor blood sugars
- Wear medical information tag
- Rx; Preg Cat C

• •

Side Effects

Headache
Weakness

Dizziness
Drowsiness

Nursing Considerations

- Management of adults with type 2 diabetes mellitus
- Do not drink alcohol since it can produce a disulfiram reaction: nausea, headache, cramps, flushing, hypoglycemia
- Assess for symptoms of cholestatic jaundice: dark urine, pruritus, yellow sclera (rare)
- Take at breakfast; onset is in 1 to 1.5 hours, peak in 1 to 3 hours, duration 10–24 hours
- Immediate-release: take 30 minutes before meals, since absorption is delayed by food
- Have a quick source of sugar or a glucagon emergency kit available
- Use sunscreen or protective clothing to prevent photosensitivity
- Extended-release tablet coating may appear in stool
- May cause hemolytic anemia when used with sulfonylurea agents in some patients
- Monitor blood sugar
- Wear medical information tag
- Rx; Preg Cat C

GLYBURIDE
(<u>glye</u>-byoo-ride)

(DiaBeta)

. . . .

METFORMIN HCL
(met-<u>for</u>-min)

(Glucophage)

Side Effects

Headache

Weakness, dizziness

GI disturbances

Allergic skin reactions

Nursing Considerations

- Management of adult type 2 diabetes mellitus
- Assess for symptoms of cholestatic jaundice: dark urine, pruritus, yellow sclera (rare)
- Take at breakfast; onset is in 2–4 hours, peak in 4 hours, duration 24 hours
- Have a quick source of sugar or a glucagon emergency kit available
- Use sunscreen or protective clothing to prevent photosensitivity
- May cause hemolytic anemia in some patients
- Monitor blood sugar
- Wear medical information tag
- Rx; Preg Cat C

• •

Side Effects

Headache

Weakness, dizziness, drowsiness

Agitation

Nausea, vomiting, diarrhea

Lactic acidosis

Flatulence

Nursing Considerations

- Management of adult type 2 diabetes mellitus
- PO: twice a day with meals to decrease GI upset and provide best absorption; may also be taken as one dose
- Can crush tablets and mix with juice or soft foods for ease of swallowing
- Do not crush, chew, or break extended-release tablet; its coating may appear in stool
- Be aware of signs of lactic acidosis: hyperventilation, fatigue, malaise, chills, myalgia, sleepiness
- Have a quick source of sugar or a glucagon emergency kit available
- Monitor blood sugar
- Off-label uses: treatment of anovulation in women with polycystic ovary syndrome
- Wear medical information tag
- Rx; Preg Cat B

PIOGLITAZONE HYDROCHLORIDE
(pye-oh-<u>gli</u>-ta-zone hahy-druh-klawr-ahyd)

(Actos)

. . . .

REPAGLINIDE
(ree-<u>pag</u>-lihn-ide)

(Prandin)

Side Effects

Cold symptoms
Headache
Sinusitis

Respiratory infection
Muscle pain
Tooth disorder

Nursing Considerations

- Treatment for type 2 diabetes
- Take around the same time each day, once daily, with or without food
- Full therapeutic effects may require 2 or more weeks
- Used in conjunction with diet and exercise regimen
- May exacerbate CHF; monitor for edema and lung sounds
- Monitor liver enzymes
- Patient should have regular eye exams for macular edema
- May increase risk of bone fractures
- Rx; Preg Cat C

• •

Side Effects

Hypoglycemia
Respiratory infection
Headache
Nausea, vomiting, diarrhea

Sinusitis
Constipation
Arthralgia
Back pain

Nursing Considerations

- Used to lower blood glucose levels in type 2 diabetes in adults
- Used in conjunction with diet and exercise regimen
- Some antifungals may inhibit metabolism
- Medication should be taken immediately before a meal
- Dose should be skipped if meal is skipped
- Do not use with NPH insulin
- Monitor blood sugar
- Rx; Preg Cat C

ROSIGLITAZONE MALEATE
(row-se-<u>glit</u>-is-own)
(Avandia)

• •

INSULIN ASPART
(NovoLog)

Side Effects

Upper respiratory infection
Headache
Back pain
Hyperglycemia

Fatigue
Bone fracture,
  especially in women

Nursing Considerations

- Used in conjunction with diet and exercise to control blood glucose levels in patients with type 2 diabetes
- Seldom used in type 1 diabetes because of the need for insulin to be present
- May be taken at any time of day without regard to meals
- Patient should be aware that rosiglitazone improves insulin sensitivity
- Liver enzyme monitoring is recommended because of hepatotoxicity possibility
- May cause heart failure in some patients
- Rx; Preg Cat C

• •

Side Effects

Hypoglycemia
Lipodystrophy
Hypokalemia
Allergic reactions

Headache
Weight gain
Edema

Nursing Considerations

- Management of diabetes in adults; the only insulin analog approved for use in external pump systems for continuous subQ insulin infusion
- Onset 15 minutes, peak 1–3 hours, duration 3–5 hours
- May be given IV under medical supervision with close blood-sugar monitoring
- Immediately follow injection with meal within 5–10 minutes
- Rx; Preg Cat B

INSULIN GLARGINE
(Lantus)

· ·

INSULIN, ISOPHANE SUSPENSION (NPH)
(Humulin N, Novolin N)

Side Effects

Hypoglycemia   Pruritus
Lipodystrophy   Rash
Allergic reactions

Nursing Considerations

- Management of diabetes in type 1 diabetics or adults with type 2 requiring a long-acting insulin to control hyperglycemia
- No pronounced peak, duration 24 hours
- Must inject at same time each day
- Not the drug of choice for diabetic ketoacidosis (use a short-acting insulin)
- Higher incidence of injection site pain compared with NPH
- Monitor blood sugar
- Do not administer IV or via insulin pump
- Do not mix with any other insulin
- Rx; Preg Cat C

• •

Side Effects

Hypoglycemia   Allergic reactions
Lipodystrophy

Nursing Considerations

- Management of diabetes
- Comes in 100 units per milliliter vial, as well as in combination with regular insulin in a 50/50 proportion and 75/25 proportion
- subQ: onset 1–1.5 hours, peak 4–12 hours, duration 18–24 hours
- Read administration instructions carefully
- Do not give IV
- Monitor blood sugar
- OTC, Rx; Preg Cat B

INSULIN LISPRO
(Humalog)

. . . .

INSULIN, REGULAR
(Humulin R)

Side Effects

Hypoglycemia   Allergic reactions
Lipodystrophy

Nursing Considerations

- Management of type 1 diabetes and in combination with sulfonylureas for type 2 diabetes
- Take within 15 minutes of eating and immediately after mixing, with combined therapy
- May be used in children in combination with sulfonylureas
- Onset rapid, peak 30 to 90 minutes, duration 6–8 hours
- May be used in an external insulin pump
- Monitor blood sugar
- If administered using insulin pen, read instructions carefully
- Do not mix with other insulins
- Available in combination with other insulin
- Rx; Preg Cat B

• •

Side Effects

Hypoglycemia   Allergic reaction
Lipodystrophy   Hypokalemia

Nursing Considerations

- Management of diabetic coma, diabetic acidosis, or other emergency conditions; esp. suitable for labile diabetes
- Comes in 100 units/milliliter vial
- Only insulin that can be given IV
- subQ: onset 30–60 minutes, peak 10–30 minutes, duration 30–60 minutes
- IV: onset 10–30 minutes, peak 10–30 minutes, duration 30–60 minutes
- Read insulin pen instructions carefully
- May be mixed with NPH *only* in same syringe; draw Novolin R first
- Do not use in insulin pumps
- Monitor blood sugar
- Do not rub after subQ injection
- OTC, Rx; Preg Cat B

GLUCAGON

(gloo-ka-gon)

(GlucaGen)

• •

ALUMINUM HYDROXIDE GEL

(Amphojel)

Side Effects

Nausea, vomiting

Nursing Considerations

- Acute management of severe hypoglycemia; facilitation of GI x-rays
- IM for hypoglycemia: onset within 10 minutes, peak 30 minutes, duration 60–90 minutes
- IV for hypoglycemia: onset within 10 minutes, peak 5 minutes, duration 60–90 minutes
- subQ for hypoglycemia: onset within 10 minutes, peak 30–45 minutes, duration 60–90 minutes
- IV for GI x-rays: onset within 45 seconds, duration dose-dependent of 9–25 minutes
- IM for GI x-rays: onset within 8–10 minutes, duration dose-dependent of 9–32 minutes
- Monitor blood sugar until patient is asymptomatic
- Use reconstituted mixture within 15 minutes of mix
- OTC, Rx; Preg Cat B

• •

Side Effects

Constipation that may   Phosphate depletion
lead to impaction

Nursing Considerations

- Antacid with duration of effect of 20 to 180 minutes
- Aluminum antacid compounds interfere with tetracycline absorption
- Contact clinician if signs of GI bleeding: tarry stools or coffee-grounds vomitus
- Shake suspension well and follow with small amount of milk or water to facilitate passage
- Monitor long-term, high-dose use if on restricted sodium intake, due to high-sodium content
- If prolonged use, monitor for phosphate depletion: anorexia, malaise, and muscle weakness; can also lead to resorption of calcium and bone demineralization in uremia patients
- Use may interfere with some imaging techniques
- Because drug contains aluminum, used in renal failure to control hyperphosphatemia by binding with phosphate in the GI tract
- Do not take longer than 2 weeks
- Rx; Preg Cat N/A

MAGALDRATE

(<u>mag</u>-al-drate)

(Riopan)

• •

CALCIUM CARBONATE

(Tums)

Side Effects

Mild constipation

Increased urine pH levels

Diarrhea

Hypophosphatemia

Nursing Considerations

- Symptomatic relief of GERD, indigestion, and GI distress
- Antacid with onset in 20 minutes and duration of 20–180 minutes
- May decrease effect of antibiotics and other drugs, such as digoxin, phenothiazines, quinidine, salicylates due to impaired absorption, so separate administration times by 1–2 hours
- Because low sodium content, used in patients on sodium restriction
- If given with enteric-coated drugs, might have premature release in stomach; separate administration times by at least 1 hour
- Shake suspension well and follow with small amount of water to facilitate passage
- Contact clinician if signs of GI bleeding: tarry stools or coffee-grounds vomitus
- Rx; Preg Cat N/A

• •

Side Effects

Nausea

Anorexia

Constipation

Dry mouth

Possible allergic reaction

Nursing Considerations

- Used as antacid and calcium supplement
- May decrease effect of some antibiotics and other drugs due to impaired absorption, so separate administration times by 2 hours
- Do not use if ventricular fibrillation or hypercalcemia
- Use caution if taking cardiac glycoside or has sarcoidosis or renal or cardiac disease
- Signs of hypercalcemia: nausea, vomiting, headache, confusion, anorexia
- OTC; Preg Cat C

DICYCLOMINE HCL
(dye-<u>sye</u>-kloh-meen)

(Bentyl)

. . . .

HYOSCYAMINE
(hye-oh-<u>sye</u>-a-meen)

(Anaspaz, Gastrosed)

Side Effects

Drowsiness
Blurred vision
Dyspnea
Dry mouth

Rash
Urinary hesitancy
Tachycardia
Headache

Nursing Considerations

- Used for treatment of irritable bowel syndrome
- Take 30 minutes before meals and at bedtime
- Use caution with potentially hazardous activities
- Report diarrhea—may be incomplete intestinal obstruction
- Rx; Preg Cat B

. . . .

Side Effects

Confusion, stimulation
  in elderly
Dry mouth, constipation
Urinary retention, hesitancy
Palpitations

Blurred vision
Tachycardia
Rash
Headache
Drowsiness

Nursing Considerations

- Treatment of peptic ulcer, other GI disorders, other spastic disorders, urinary incontinence
- PO: onset 20–30 minutes, duration 4–6 hours
- IM, IV, subQ: onset 2–3 minutes, duration 4–6 hours
- Avoid activities requiring alertness until stabilized on med
- Avoid alcohol, CNS depressants
- Use sunglasses to prevent photophobia
- Take 30–60 minutes before meals
- Avoid antacids within 1 hour
- Rx; Preg Cat C

LOPERAMIDE HCL
(loe-<u>per</u>-a-mide)

(Imodium)

• •

MECLIZINE
(<u>mek</u>-li-zeen)

(Antivert, Bonine)

Side Effects

Nausea, vomiting
Abdominal pain/distention
Dizziness

Drowsiness
Dry mouth

Nursing Considerations

- Used for control of diarrhea, including diarrhea in travelers
- Take with a full glass of water
- Encourage 6 to 8 glasses of fluid per day
- Use caution with potentially hazardous activities
- If abdominal distention in acute ulcerative colitis, stop med
- Avoid use with alcohol, CNS depressants
- Follow clear liquid or bland diet until diarrhea subsides
- Do not use OTC if fever over 101°F (38°C) or if bloody diarrhea
- OTC, Rx; Preg Cat C

• •

Side Effects

Drowsiness
Dizziness

Nursing Considerations

- Management of vertigo, motion sickness
- Duration 8–14 hours
- Take 1 hour before traveling
- Avoid activities requiring alertness
- Avoid alcohol, CNS depressants
- OTC, Rx; Preg Cat B

METOCLOPRAMIDE HCL
(met-oh-<u>kloe</u>-pra-mide)

(Reglan)

. . . .

PROCHLORPERAZINE
(proe-klor-<u>pair</u>-a-zeen)

(Compro)

Side Effects

Drowsiness
Restlessness
Lassitude
Headache

Sleeplessness
Dry mouth
Anxiety

Nursing Considerations

- Prevention of nausea, vomiting induced by chemotherapy, radiation, delayed gastric emptying, GERD
- Used with tube feeding to decrease residual and risk of aspiration
- PO: take 30–60 minutes before meals or procedures
- IV: inject slowly over 1–2 minutes; infuse over 15 minutes
- Use caution with potentially hazardous activities
- Avoid alcohol, CNS depressants
- May cause tardive dyskinesia
- May cause depression
- Rx; Preg Cat B

• •

Side Effects

Orthostatic hypotension
Blurred vision
Dry eyes, dry mouth

Constipation
Drowsiness
Photosensitivity

Nursing Considerations

- Management of nausea, vomiting, psychotic disorders
- Monitor for development of neuroleptic malignant syndrome (fever, respiratory distress, tachycardia, convulsions, sweating, hypertension or hypotension, pallor, tiredness, severe muscle stiffness, loss of bladder control); notify clinician immediately
- PO: take with food
- Do not crush or break sustained-release capsules
- IM: inject slowly, deeply into gluteal UOQ; keep patient lying down for 30 minutes
- Use caution with potentially hazardous activities
- Avoid changing positions (lying/sitting/standing) rapidly
- Wear sunscreen and protective clothing to prevent photosensitivity reactions
- Check CBC and liver functions with prolonged use
- Risk of increase mortality in elderly patients with dementia; related psychosis
- May develop tardive dyskinesia
- Rx; Preg Cat C

PROMETHAZINE
(pro-<u>meth</u>-a-zeen)

(Phenergan)

• •

SIMETHICONE
(si-<u>meth</u>-i-kone)

Side Effects

Drowsiness
Dizziness
Constipation

Urinary retention
Dry mouth
Hyperglycemia

Nursing Considerations

- Management of motion sickness, rhinitis, allergy symptoms, sedation, nausea, pre- and postoperative sedation
- PO: onset 20 minutes, duration 4–6 hours
- Take 30–60 minutes before traveling
- Avoid activities requiring alertness
- Avoid alcohol, CNS depressants
- May cause severe chemical irritation and damage to tissue
- May lower seizure threshold
- May cause false results in pregnancy testing
- Rx; Preg Cat C

• •

Side Effects

Belching
Rectal flatus

Nursing Considerations

- Helps disperse gas pockets in GI system, does not decrease gas production
- Take after meals, at bedtime
- Shake suspension well before pouring
- Tablets must be chewed
- OTC, Rx; Preg Cat C

ESOMEPRAZOLE MAGNESIUM
(e-sew-<u>mep</u>-ruh-zole)

(Nexium)

· ·

OMEPRAZOLE
(oh-<u>meh</u>-pruh-zole)

(Prilosec)

Side Effects

Headache
Diarrhea
Nausea

Flatulence
Dry mouth

Nursing Considerations

- Short-term treatment of erosive esophagitis
- Used to treat GERD
- Take at least 60 minutes before meals
- Swallow capsules whole, do not chew
- May be taken in conjunction with antacids
- Rx; Preg Cat B

• •

Side Effects

Headache
Nausea, vomiting, diarrhea

Flatulence

Nursing Considerations

- Treatment of active duodenal ulcers
- Treatment of GERD in patients over age 2 years
- Take 30 minutes before eating
- May be taken at the same time as antacids
- OTC, Rx; Preg Cat C

CIMETIDINE
(sye-<u>met</u>-ih-deen)

(Tagamet)

FAMOTIDINE
(fa-<u>moe</u>-ti-deen)

(Pepcid)

Side Effects

Diarrhea
Confusion (esp. in elderly
    with large doses)

Headache
Dysrhythmias

Nursing Considerations

- Treatment of chronic warts in children
- Reduces gastric acid secretions by 50%–80%
- May be taken without regard to meals
- Avoid antacids 1 hour before or after dose
- Do not use OTC for more than 2 weeks unless medically
  supervised
- Monitor liver enzymes and blood counts
- May be used for prevention of aspiration pneumonia, stress
  ulcers, idiopathic urticaria, hyperparathyroidism
- OTC, Rx; Preg Cat B

• •

Side Effects

Headache
Blood dyscrasias
Hepatitis

Dizziness
Constipation

Nursing Considerations

- Treatment of duodenal and gastric ulcers, GERD, heartburn
- PO: onset 30–60 minutes, peak 1–3 hours, duration 6–12 hours
- IV: onset immediate, peak 30–60 minutes, duration 8–15 hours
- Signs of blood dyscrasia: bleeding, bruising, fatigue, malaise,
  poor healing, jaundice
- OTC, Rx; Preg Cat B

LANSOPRAZOLE
(lan-<u>so</u>-prey-zohl)

(Prevacid)

· ·

MISOPROSTOL
(mis-oh-<u>prost</u>-ole)

(Cytotec)

Side Effects

Dizziness   Abdominal pain
Diarrhea

Nursing Considerations

- Used for treatment of GERD and ulcers, erosive esophagitis
- PO: take no more than 30 minutes before meals; capsules may be opened and sprinkled on food (applesauce, pudding, cottage cheese, yogurt) and swallowed immediately
- Can use with antacids
- Do not crush or chew capsule contents
- To give with NG tube in place, open the capsule and mix with orange, apple or tomato juice, instill through NG tube and flush with additional juice to clear tube
- Report severe diarrhea
- Rx; Preg Cat B

• •

Side Effects

Abdominal pain   Nausea
Diarrhea   Headache
Miscarriage

Nursing Considerations

- Prevention of gastric ulcers during NSAID therapy
- Take with meals and at bedtime
- Avoid taking magnesium antacids within 2 hours
- Notify clinician if diarrhea lasts more than 1 week
- Notify clinician if black, tarry stools or severe abdominal pain
- Rx; Preg Cat X

RABEPRAZOLE
(rah-<u>bep</u>-rah-zole)

(AcipHex)

• •

RANITIDINE
(ra-<u>nit</u>-i-deen)

(Zantac)

Side Effects

Headache

Dizziness

Nausea, vomiting, diarrhea

Constipation, flatulence

Rash

Back pain

Nursing Considerations

- Used for treatment of GERD and duodenal ulcers
- Take on an empty stomach before eating
- Swallow tablets whole; do not crush, chew, or split tablets
- Avoid alcohol, NSAIDs, and ASA; may increase gastric upset
- Rx; Preg Cat B

• •

Side Effects

Dizziness (esp. in elderly)

Drowsiness

Headache

Nursing Considerations

- Used to inhibit gastric acid secretion, ulcers (GI)
- Take with or immediately following meals
- Do not take antacids within 1 hour before or after
- Do not smoke; it interferes with healing and drug's effectiveness
- Avoid alcohol, ASA, and caffeine, which increase stomach acid
- False positive tests for urine protein may occur
- OTC, Rx; Preg Cat B

SUCRALFATE
(soo-<u>kral</u>-fate)

(Carafate)

· ·

SULFASALAZINE
(sul-fah-<u>sal</u>-ah-zeen)

(Azulfidine)

Side Effects

Constipation
Hypersensitivity

Nursing Considerations

- Short-term treatment (less than 8 weeks) of duodenal ulcers
- PO: 1 hour before meals or 2 hours after meals and at bedtime with full glass of water
- Do not chew tablets
- Do not use antacids within 30 minutes of med
- Encourage 8 to 10 glasses of fluid per day
- Avoid smoking
- Rx; Preg Cat B

. . . .

Side Effects

Headache   Fever
Anorexia   Oligospermia
Nausea, vomiting, diarrhea   Hepatotoxicity
Rashes

Nursing Considerations

- Used for treatment of inflammatory bowel diseases and arthritis
- PO: take with food to decrease GI upset
- Encourage fluids to decrease crystallization in kidneys
- May permanently stain contact lens yellow
- May cause orange-yellow urine and skin, which is not significant
- Wear sunscreen and protective clothing to prevent photosensitivity reactions
- Monitor liver enzymes
- Rx; Preg Cat B

PHENTERMINE
(<u>fen</u>-ter-meen)

(Ionamin)

• •

SIBUTRAMINE
(sih-<u>byoo</u>-truh-mine)

(Meridia)

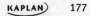

Side Effects

CNS stimulation
Hypertension
Changes in libido

Palpitations
Drowsiness

Nursing Considerations

- Short-term treatment of obesity
- PO: hydrochloride form duration is 4 hours
- PO: resin complex form duration is 12–14 hours
- Take 30 minutes before meals or as a single dose before breakfast or 10–14 hours before bedtime
- Avoid activities requiring alertness until response is known
- Avoid alcohol, CNS depressants
- Contact clinician if chest pain, decreased exercise tolerance, fainting, or lower extremity swelling
- Controlled Substance Schedule IV; Preg Cat C

• •

Side Effects

Headache
Dry mouth
Anorexia
Constipation
Insomnia

Rhinitis
Back pain
Hypertension
Tachycardia
Migraine

Nursing Considerations

- Used to manage weight loss and maintenance in obesity
- Should be used with a reduced-calorie diet
- Regular heart rate and blood pressure monitoring is important
- Avoid use with MAOIs
- Should not be used in patients with cardiac disease
- Rx C-IV; Preg Cat C

LACTULOSE SYRUP
(<u>lak</u>-tyoo-lose)

(Enulose)

• •

PANCREATIN
(<u>pan</u>-kree-a-tin)

Side Effects
Nausea, vomiting
Abdominal cramps

Nursing Considerations
- Used for chronic constipation; prevention and treatment of portal-systemic encephalotic including hepatic precoma and coma
- PO: take with water or fruit juice to counteract sweet taste
- Use with caution in diabetics
- Monitor blood sugar
- Rx; Preg Cat B

• •

Side Effects
Anorexia	Constipation
Nausea, vomiting, diarrhea	Hives

Nursing Considerations
- Do not crush or break enteric-coated capsules
- Do not use if sensitive or allergy to pork
- OTC, Rx: Preg Cat C

PANCRELIPASE

(pan-kree-<u>ly</u>-payz)

(Pancrease, Viokase)

· ·

TAMSULOSIN HYDROCHLORIDE

(tam-sull-<u>oh</u>-sin hahy-druh-klawr-ahyd)

(Flomax)

Side Effects

Abdominal pain
  (high doses only)
Nausea, diarrhea
Stomach cramps

Flatulence
Abnormal feces
Fatigue

Nursing Considerations

- Used to replace or supplement naturally occurring enzymes; contains lipase, amylase, and protease lost due to cystic fibrosis
- Take with 8 ounces of water and food, swallow right away, sit up when taking
- Do not crush or break enteric-coated capsules
- Do not use if sensitive or allergy to pork
- Stools will be foul-smelling and frothy
- Rx; Preg Cat C

• •

Side Effects

Sleepiness, difficulty falling
  or staying asleep
Weakness
Back pain
Nausea, vomiting, diarrhea
UTI
Cold symptoms, including
  pain or pressure in the face

Blurred vision
Abnormal ejaculation
Dizziness
Headache
Increased cough
Chest pain
Priapism

Nursing Considerations

- Treatment of benign prostatic hyperplasia
- Take the same time daily, once a day, 30 minutes after a meal
- Avoid changing positions (lying, sitting, standing) rapidly
- Use caution in potentially hazardous activities
- May have cross-allergy with sulfa drugs
- This medication should be stopped prior to cataract surgery; may cause IFIS
- Rx; Preg Cat B

OXYBUTYNIN CHLORIDE
(ox-i-<u>byoo</u>-ti-nin)
(Ditropan)

• •

TOLTERODINE TARTRATE
(toal-<u>tear</u>-oh-dene)
(Detrol, Detrol LA)

Side Effects

Anxiety, restlessness
Dizziness
Convulsions
Palpitations, tachycardia
Drowsiness, blurred vision

Nausea, vomiting
Anorexia
Dry mouth
Mydriasis
Constipation

Nursing Considerations

- Antispasmodic treatment of neurogenic bladder
- Take on an empty stomach
- Avoid alcohol, CNS depressants
- Avoid activities requiring alertness until med response is known
- Decreased ability to perspire; avoid strenuous activity in warm weather
- Wear sunglasses in bright sunlight to prevent photophobia
- Rx; Preg Cat B

• •

Side Effects

Dry mouth
Dizziness
Constipation

Dyspepsia
Somnolence
Blurred vision

Nursing Considerations

- Used to treat patients with overactive bladder
- Effective with frequency, urgency, or incontinence symptoms
- Patients should avoid alcohol during treatment with tolterodine
- Missed doses should be skipped, return to normal schedule
- Rx; Preg Cat C

SILDENAFIL CITRATE
(sil-<u>den</u>-a-fill)

(Viagra)

• •

TADALAFIL
(teh-<u>dal</u>-uh-fil)

(Cialis)

Side Effects

Headache, flushing
Dizziness
Upset stomach
Nasal congestion
UTI

Abnormal vision
Rash
Tinnitus, hearing loss
Visual disturbances

Nursing Considerations

- Treatment of erectile dysfunction
- Take approximately 1 hour before sexual activity
- Do not use more than once a day
- Tablets may be split
- High-fat meal will reduce absorption; better absorption on empty stomach
- Never use with nitrates; could have fatal fall in blood pressure
- Notify clinician if erection lasts longer than 4 hours
- Stop medication if hearing or visual disturbances occur
- Rx; Preg Cat B

• •

Side Effects

Headache
Dyspepsia
Back pain

Tinnitus, hearing loss
Myalgia
Nasal congestion

Nursing Considerations

- Used to treat erectile dysfunction
- Patients with severe hepatic impairment should not take Tadalafil
- Contraindicated in patients taking nitrates or alpha-adrenergic blockers
- Tadalafil does not protect against sexually transmitted diseases
- Alert physician if erection lasts more than 4 hours
- Stop medication if hearing or visual disturbances occur
- Alcohol intake may increase orthostatic symptoms
- Rx; Preg Cat B

VARDENAFIL
(var-<u>den</u>-uh-fil)

(Levitra)

• •

FINASTERIDE
(fin-<u>as</u>-teh-ride)

(Proscar, Propecia)

Side Effects

Headache
Nasal congestion
Flushing

Dyspepsia
Tinnitus, hearing loss

Nursing Considerations

- Used to treat erectile dysfunction
- Contraindicated in patients taking organic nitrates
- Contact physician if erection lasts over 4 hours
- Plasma levels peak in 30 minutes to 2 hours
- Stop medication if hearing or visual disturbances occur
- Alpha blocker used with this medication may cause syncope
- Rx; Preg Cat B

• •

Side Effects

Decreased libido
Decreased volume of
  ejaculate
Testicular pain

Impotence
Breast tenderness and
  enlargement
Angioedema

Nursing Considerations

- Treatment of BPH by Proscar, male hair loss by Propecia
- May be taken without regard for food
- Pregnant women should avoid contact with crushed drug or
  patient's semen; may adversely affect developing male fetus
- Full therapeutic effect: Propecia may require 3 months, Proscar
  may require 6–12 months
- Not for use in women and children
- Rx; Preg Cat X

PHENAZOPYRIDINE HCL
(fen-az-oh-<u>peer</u>-i-deen)

(Pyridium)

. . . .

Genitourinary Medications
Urinary Anti-Infectives

NITROFURANTOIN
(nye-troe-<u>fyoor</u>-an-toyn)

(Furadantin, Macrobid, Macrodantin)

Side Effects

GI upset

Kidney and liver toxicity

Rash

Headache

Nursing Considerations

- Treatment of urinary tract irritation, often paired with urinary anti-infective
- Do not crush tablets; can take with food or milk to decrease GI upset
- Inform patient that urine will be bright orange/red
- Monitor for signs of hepatoxicity: dark urine, clay-colored stools, jaundice, itching, abdominal pain, fever, diarrhea
- May interfere with urine glucose tests
- OTC, Rx; Preg Cat B

• •

Side Effects

Dizziness

Nausea, vomiting, diarrhea

Abdominal pain

Tooth staining

Hypersensitivity

Nursing Considerations

- Treatment of UTIs
- Take with food or milk
- Avoid alcohol
- Two daily doses if urine output is high or patient has diabetes
- Drug may turn urine rust-yellow to brown
- May cause false positive glucose in urine
- May increase AST and ALT
- Rx; Preg Cat B

ALENDRONATE
(al-en-<u>drone</u>-ate)

(Fosamax)

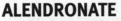

RISEDRONATE
(riss-<u>ed</u>-roe-nate)

(Actonel)

Side Effects

Esophageal ulceration   Musculoskeletal pain
GI distress

Nursing Considerations

- Prevention and treatment of osteoporosis in women; treatment of osteoporosis in men; treatment of Paget disease
- Onset: 1 month, peak 3–6 months, duration 3 weeks to 7 months
- Take in A.M. before food or other meds with full glass of water; remain upright for 30 minutes
- If dose missed, skip dose; do not double dose or take later in the day
- Take with calcium and vitamin D if instructed by clinician
- May cause atypical subtrochanteric femur fractures
- Rx; Preg Cat C

• •

Side Effects

Weakness   Joint pain
Diarrhea, abdominal pain   Dyspepsia
Bone pain   Hypersensitivity
Back pain   Eye inflammation

Nursing Considerations

- Prevention and treatment of osteoporosis in women; treatment of osteoporosis in men; treatment of Paget disease
- Onset: within days, peak 30 days, duration up to 16 months
- Take in A.M. before food or other meds with full glass of water; remain upright for 30 minutes
- Take with calcium and vitamin D if instructed by clinician
- May cause atypical subtrochanteric femur fractures
- Rx; Preg Cat C

ETIDRONATE
(eh-tih-<u>droe</u>-nate)

(Didronel)

• •

Hormones/Synthetic Substitutes/Modifiers
Thyroid Hormones

THYROID, DESICCATED
(<u>thigh</u>-roid)

(Armour Thyroid)

Side Effects

Nausea, diarrhea	Hypersensitivity
Bone pain and tenderness	Headache
Myalgia	Arthralgia

Nursing Considerations

- Treatment of Paget disease, used with total hip replacement and spinal cord injury, hyperkalemia of cancer
- PO: onset 1 month, duration 1 year
- IV: onset 24 hours, peak 3 days, duration 11 days
- Take on empty stomach with calcium and vitamin D, but not within 2 hours of med
- Contact clinician if sudden onset of unexpected pain, restricted mobility, heat over bone
- May cause atypical subtrochanteric femur fractures
- Rx; Preg Cat C

• •

Side Effects

Weight loss	Tachycardia
Palpitations	Sweating
Diarrhea	

Nursing Considerations

- Used to treat adult hypothyroidism
- Side effects are rare and generally associated with overdosing
- Dosed at 15–30 mg initially and titrated up every 2–3 weeks until optimum results are present
- Thyroid levels should be checked every 6 months after patient is stabilized
- Patient should avoid OTC preparations and food with iodine
- Rx; Preg Cat A

LEVOTHYROXINE (T4)
(lee-voe-thye-<u>rox</u>-een)

(Synthroid, Levothroid)

· ·

Mental Health Medications
Antianxiety Agents

ALPRAZOLAM
(al-<u>pray</u>-zoe-lam)

(Xanax)

Side Effects

Weight loss

Arrhythmias, tachycardia

Insomnia, irritability

Nervousness

Heat intolerance

Menstrual irregularities

Nursing Considerations

- Management of hypothyroidism, myxedema coma, thyroid hormone replacement
- PO: peak 1–3 weeks, duration 1–3 weeks
- IV: onset 6–8 hours, peak 24 hours
- PO: take at same time daily to maintain blood level; take on empty stomach
- Do not switch brands unless directed
- Avoid OTC meds with iodine and iodized salt, soybeans, tofu, turnips, walnuts, some seafood, some bread
- Drug is not a cure, but controls symptoms and treatment is lifelong
- Rx; Preg Cat A

• •

Side Effects

Dizziness, drowsiness

Orthostatic hypotension

Blurred vision

Nursing Considerations

- Management of anxiety, panic disorders, premenstrual dysphoric disorders
- Onset 30 minutes, peak 1–2 hours, duration 4–6 hours
- Full therapeutic response takes 2 to 3 days
- May be taken with food
- May be habit-forming; do not take for longer than 4 months unless directed
- Memory impairment is a sign of long-term use
- Do not stop drug abruptly; may cause seizures
- Drowsiness may worsen at beginning of treatment
- May produce emotional and/or physical dependence
- Rx; Preg Cat D

BUSPIRONE
(byoo-<u>spye</u>-rone)

(BuSpar)

. . . .

CHLORDIAZEPOXIDE
(klor-dye-az-e-<u>pox</u>-ide)

(Librium)

Side Effects

Dizziness, headache
Stimulation, insomnia,
  nervousness

Light-headedness, numbness
Nausea, diarrhea, constipation
Tachycardia, palpitations

Nursing Considerations

- Management of anxiety disorders
- Onset 7–10 days, optimum effect may take 3–4 weeks
- Use caution with activities requiring alertness until response to med is known
- Avoid alcohol, CNS depressants, and large amounts of grapefruit juice
- Use caution when changing positions because fainting may occur, especially in elderly
- Drowsiness may worsen at beginning of treatment
- Rx; Preg Cat B

• •

Side Effects

Dizziness
Drowsiness
Pain at IM site

Ataxia
Disorientation

Nursing Considerations

- Management of anxiety and treatment of alcohol withdrawal, IBS
- PO: onset 1–2 hours, peak 30 minutes to 4 hours
- IM: onset 15–30 minutes, slow, erratic absorption
- IV: onset 1–5 minutes, duration 15–60 minutes
- Use caution with activities requiring alertness until response to med is known
- Abrupt stop may lead to withdrawal: insomnia, irritability, nervousness, tremors
- Avoid alcohol, CNS depressants
- Tablets may be crushed and taken with food or fluids for ease of swallowing
- Rx; C-IV; Preg Cat D

DIAZEPAM
(dye-<u>az</u>-e-pam)
(Valium)

. . . .

LORAZEPAM
(lor-<u>a</u>-ze-pam)
(Ativan)

Side Effects

Drowsiness, fatigue, ataxia

Hypotension

Paradoxic anxiety, esp. in elderly

Orthostatic hypotension

Blurred vision

Nursing Considerations

- Treatment of anxiety, acute alcohol withdrawal, seizures; skeletal muscle relaxant; preoperative medication
- PO: may be taken with food, onset 30 minutes
- IM: inject deep, slowly into large muscle mass; onset 15–30 minutes, duration 60–90 minutes, slow and erratic absorption
- IV: into large vein, push doses should not exceed 5 mg/minute, resuscitation equipment available; onset immediate, duration 15 minutes to 1 hour
- Smoking may decrease effectiveness
- Avoid use with alcohol, CNS depressants
- Long-term use withdrawal symptoms: vomiting, sweating, abdominal/muscle cramps, tremors, and possibly convulsions
- May be habit-forming if used over 4 months
- Rx; C-IV; Preg Cat D

• •

Side Effects

Dizziness, drowsiness

Orthostatic hypotension

Blurred vision

Weakness

Disorientation

Visual disturbance

Nursing Considerations

- Treatment of anxiety, irritability in psychiatric or organic disorders; treatment of insomnia; adjunct in endoscopic procedures; preoperative medication
- PO: onset 30 minutes, peak 1–6 hours
- IM: onset 15–30 minutes, peak 60–90 minutes
- IV: onset 5–15 minutes, peak unknown
- May be taken with food
- May be habit-forming; do not take for longer than 4 months unless directed
- Avoid alcohol, CNS depressants
- Do not stop drug abruptly
- Drowsiness may worsen at beginning of treatment
- Rx; Preg Cat C-IV

CITALOPRAM
(sit-<u>al</u>-oh-pram)

(Celexa)

· ·

ESCITALOPRAM OXALATE
(es-sye-<u>tal</u>-oh-pram)

(Lexapro)

Side Effects

Palpitations, tachycardia

Nausea, vomiting, diarrhea

Decreased appetite

Nervousness, insomnia

Drowsiness

Hyponatremia

Nursing Considerations

- Treatment of major depression
- Take in A.M. to avoid insomnia
- Can potentiate effects of digoxin, warfarin, and diazepam
- Avoid use with alcohol, CNS depressants for up to 1 week after end of therapy
- Use caution in potentially hazardous activities
- Avoid changing positions (lying, sitting, standing) rapidly
- Take consistently at same time of day; therapeutic effects in up to 4 weeks
- May increase risk of suicidal thoughts and behavior
- Rx; Preg Cat C

- -

Side Effects

Nausea, diarrhea, constipation

Insomnia

Fatigue, drowsiness

Decreased libido, sexual dysfunction

Increased sweating

Increased appetite, heartburn, stomach pain

Flulike symptoms, runny nose, sneezing

Dry mouth

Dizziness

Labile blood sugar

Hypokalemia

Hyponatremia

Visual disturbances

Nursing Considerations

- Treatment of major depression, anxiety
- Take consistently at same time of day; full therapeutic effect may require 4 weeks
- May require gradual reduction before stopping
- Can potentiate effects of digoxin, warfarin, diazepam
- Use caution in potentially hazardous activities; avoid use with alcohol
- May increase risk of suicidal thoughts or behaviors
- Monitor for SIADH
- Teach patient to avoid aspirin and NSAIDs due to increased bleeding risk
- May cause serotonin syndrome or NMS; monitor for change in mental status, hyperthermia, tachycardia, labile BP, and incoordination
- Rx; Preg Cat C

FLUOXETINE HCL
(floo-<u>ox</u>-uh-teen)

(Prozac)

• •

PAROXETINE HCL
(pair-<u>ox</u>-eh-teen)

(Paxil)

Side Effects

Palpitations

Nausea, diarrhea, constipation

Decreased appetite with
significant weight loss

Nervousness, insomnia

Urinary retention

Drowsiness

Rash, pruritus, excessive
sweating

Fatigue

Nursing Considerations

- Treatment of depression/OCD, bulimia, PMDD
- Take consistently at same time of day; full therapeutic effects
  may require 4 weeks
- Can potentiate effects of digoxin, warfarin, diazepam, NSAID,
  and aspirin
- Used for anorexia, not suicidal or homicidal emotions
- Avoid use with alcohol, CNS depressants for up to 1 week after
  end of therapy
- Use caution in potentially hazardous activities
- May increase risk of suicidal thoughts or behavior
- Rx; Preg Cat C

• •

Side Effects

Palpitations

Nausea, vomiting, diarrhea,
constipation

Hyponatremia

Decreased appetite

Nervousness, insomnia

Nursing Considerations

- Treatment of anxiety, depression, OCD and social anxiety
  disorder, panic disorder, PTSD
- Take consistently at same time of day; therapeutic effects in up
  to 4 weeks
- Do not chew or crush
- May increase risk of suicidal thoughts or behavior
- May increase risk for bleeding
- Avoid use with alcohol, CNS depressants for up to 1 week after
  end of therapy
- Use caution in potentially hazardous activities
- Rx; Preg Cat D

SERTRALINE HCL
(<u>sir</u>-trah-leen)

(Zoloft)

· ·

Mental Health Medications
Antidepressants, Tricyclic

AMITRIPTYLINE
(a-mee-<u>trip</u>-ti-leen)

Side Effects

Headache

Dizziness

Tremor

Nausea, diarrhea

Insomnia

Dry mouth

Male sexual dysfunction

Nursing Considerations

- Treatment of depression, OCD, panic disorder with or without agoraphobia, PTSD, PMDD, and social phobia
- Take consistently at same time of day; therapeutic effects take up to 4 weeks
- Can potentiate effects of digoxin, warfarin, diazepam, aspirin, and NSAIDs
- Used for anorexia, not suicidal or homicidal emotions
- Avoid use with alcohol, CNS depressants for up to 1 week after end of therapy; avoid disulfiram
- Use caution in potentially hazardous activities
- May increase risk of suicidal thoughts or behavior
- Rx, Preg Cat C

• •

Side Effects

Sedation/drowsiness

Blurred vision, dry mouth, diaphoresis

Postural hypotension, palpitations

Nausea, vomiting, diarrhea

Constipation, urinary retention

Increased appetite

Sexual dysfunction

Confusion

Cardiac dysrhythmias

Nursing Considerations

- Treatment of major depression
- Suicide risk high after 10–14 days due to increased energy
- Avoid use with alcohol
- Sunblock required
- Increase fluid intake
- Take dose at bedtime due to sedative effect
- Heavy smokers may require a larger dose
- Use safety precautions with hazardous activity
- Avoid sudden positional changes, partial hypotension
- Blood sugar may be altered; monitor blood sugar in diabetic patients
- Rx; Preg Cat C

DOXEPIN
(<u>dox</u>-e-pin)

• •

IMIPRAMINE
(im-<u>ip</u>-ra-meen)

(Tofranil)

Side Effects

Sedation/drowsiness

Blurred vision, dry mouth, diaphoresis

Postural hypotension, palpitations

Nausea, vomiting, diarrhea

Constipation, urinary retention

Anorexia

Sexual dysfunction

Nursing Considerations

- Psychoneurotic patient with depression and or anxiety; hypnotic for insomnia
- Avoid use with alcohol
- Suicide risk high after 10–14 day due to increased energy
- Increase fluid intake
- Take dose at bedtime due to sedative effect
- Heavy smokers may require a larger dose
- Use safety precautions with hazardous activity
- Avoid sudden positional changes
- May cause "sleep" activities such as driving a car, eating, communicating with others
- May worsen depression
- Rx; Preg Cat C

● ●

Side Effects

Sedation/drowsiness

Dry mouth

Postural hypotension, palpitations

Diarrhea

Urinary retention

Anorexia

Confusion

Nursing Considerations

- Psychoneurotic patient with depression and anxiety; hypnotic for insomnia
- Full therapeutic effect may take 2–3 weeks
- Drug is dispensed in small amounts at beginning of treatment due to suicide potential
- Use safety precautions with hazardous activity
- Avoid sudden positional changes
- Do not stop abruptly: could cause nausea, malaise, headache
- Avoid alcohol, CNS depressants
- Rx; Preg Cat C

NORTRIPTYLINE

(nor-<u>trip</u>-ti-leen)

(Pamelor)

• •

BUPROPION HCL

(byoo-<u>proe</u>-pee-on)

**(Wellbutrin, Wellbutrin SR,
Wellbutrin XL, Zyban)**

Side Effects

Sedation/drowsiness
Blurred vision, dry mouth, diaphoresis
Postural hypotension, palpitations

Nausea, vomiting, diarrhea
Constipation, urinary retention
Increased appetite
Sexual dysfunction

Nursing Considerations

- Treatment of major depression
- Avoid use with alcohol, CNS depressants
- Suicide risk high after 10–14 days due to increased energy
- Increase fluid intake
- Take dose at bedtime due to sedative effect
- Heavy smokers may require a larger dose
- Use safety precautions with hazardous activity
- Avoid sudden positional changes, partial hypotension
- Women: avoid use if pregnant, breastfeeding
- Rx; Preg Cat C

• •

Side Effects

Agitation
Nausea, vomiting
Headache
Dry mouth

Tremor
Hypertension
Insomnia
Nervousness

Nursing Considerations

- Treatment of depression and smoking cessation
- If missed dose for depression, take as soon as possible and space remaining doses at not less than 4-hour intervals
- If missed dose for smoking cessation, omit dose
- May require gradual reduction before stopping
- Avoid use with alcohol, CNS depressants for up to 1 week after end of therapy
- Use caution in potentially hazardous activities
- Avoid changing positions (lying, sitting, standing) rapidly
- May increase risk for suicidal thoughts or behavior
- Rx; Preg Cat B

DULOXETINE HYDROCHLORIDE
(doo-<u>lox</u>-e-teen hahy-druh-klawr-ahyd)

(Cymbalta)

. . . .

MIRTAZAPINE
(mer-<u>taz</u>-e-peen)

(Remeron)

Side Effects

Nausea, vomiting, diarrhea, constipation

Decreased appetite, stomach pain

Heartburn

Dry mouth

Increased urination, difficulty urinating

Dizziness, headache

Tiredness, weakness, drowsiness

Muscle pain or cramps

Increased sweating, night sweats

Sexual dysfunction

Uncontrollable shaking of a part of the body

Nursing Considerations

- Treatment of depression, anxiety, diabetic neuropathy, and fibromyalgia
- Take the same time daily, once or twice a day for depression; once a day for anxiety, diabetic neuropathy, or fibromyalgia; full therapeutic effects may require 4 weeks
- May require gradual reduction before stopping
- Avoid changing positions (lying, sitting, standing) rapidly
- Avoid use with alcohol
- Use caution in potentially hazardous activities
- May increase risk of suicidal thoughts or behaviors
- Teach patient to avoid aspirin and NSAIDs due to increased bleeding risk
- Monitor BP
- Monitor blood sugar in diabetics; may cause hyperglycemia
- Rx; Preg Cat C

• •

Side Effects

Drowsiness, dizziness

Increased appetite, weight gain

Constipation

Dry mouth

Somnolence

Nursing Considerations

- Treatment of depression
- Do not use within 14 days of MAOI
- May require gradual reduction before stopping
- Check with clinician before taking OTC cold remedy
- Avoid use with alcohol, CNS depressants for up to 1 week after end of therapy
- Use caution in potentially hazardous activities
- May increase risk for suicidal thoughts or behavior
- Rx; Preg Cat C

TRAZODONE
(<u>tray</u>-zoe-doan)

• •

VENLAFAXINE
(ven-lah-<u>fax</u>-een)

(Effexor, Effexor XR)

Side Effects

Drowsiness	Dizziness	Blurred vision
Hypotension	Priapism	Constipation
Dry mouth	Hyponatremia	
Nausea	Somnolence	

Nursing Considerations

- Treatment of major depression
- Take with or immediately after meals to lessen GI upset
- If dose missed, take immediately, unless within 4 hours of next dose
- May require gradual reduction before stopping
- Avoid use with alcohol, CNS depressants for up to 1 week after end of therapy
- Use caution in potentially hazardous activities
- Avoid changing positions (lying, sitting, standing) rapidly
- May increase risk of suicidal thoughts or behavior
- Take at same time, preferably at bedtime on empty stomach
- Rx; Preg Cat C

● ●

Side Effects

Abnormal dreams, insomnia	Abdominal pain	Sedation
Anxiety, nervousness	Nausea, vomiting, diarrhea	Mydriasis
Dizziness, weakness	Anorexia, weight loss	Hypertension
Headache	Sexual dysfunction	Serotonin syndrome

Nursing Considerations

- Treatment of major depression or relapse, generalized anxiety disorder
- Take with food; extended-release tablets should be swallowed whole
- If dose is missed, take immediately unless time for next dose
- May require gradual reduction before stopping if taken over 6 weeks
- Avoid use with alcohol, CNS depressants for up to 1 week after end of therapy
- Use caution in potentially hazardous activities
- Avoid changing positions (lying, sitting, standing) rapidly
- May increase risk of suicidal thoughts or behavior
- May increase risk of GI bleed
- Rx; Preg Cat C

HALOPERIDOL
(ha-loe-<u>per</u>-i-dole)
(Haldol)

• •

OLANZAPINE
(oh-<u>lan</u>-zuh-peen)
(Zyprexa)

Side Effects

Drowsiness	Tachycardia	Dystonia
Dizziness	Hypotension	Hyperpyrexia
Hallucinations	Confusion	Schizophrenia
Tardive dyskinesia	Hypertension	

Nursing Considerations

- Treatment of Tourette syndrome, schizophrenia
- PO concentrate: dilute with water, not coffee or tea
- PO: take with food or full glass of water/milk
- IM: inject slowly, deep into UOQ of buttock; have patient lie down for 30 minutes; do not give IV
- Avoid abrupt withdrawal; discontinue gradually
- Avoid use with alcohol, CNS depressants
- Use caution in potentially hazardous activities
- Avoid changing positions (lying/sitting/standing) rapidly
- Wear protective clothing, sunglasses due to photosensitivity
- Rx; Preg Cat C

• •

Side Effects

Somnolence	Nervousness	Increase appetite
Agitation	Joint pain	and weight gain
Hostility	Dry mouth	Fatigue
Dizziness	Headache	
Rhinitis	Insomnia	

Nursing Considerations

- Useful in schizophrenia and bipolar I disorder
- Has been used successfully in manic episodes associated with bipolar I
- Use caution when rising due to postural hypotension possibility
- Dosage should be managed tightly when established
- Use caution when operating equipment
- Monitor weight
- Monitor blood glucose in diabetic patients; may cause hyperglycemia
- Rx; Preg Cat C

RISPERIDONE
(riss-<u>pair</u>-i-doan)

(Risperdal)

· ·

QUETIAPINE
(kweh-<u>tie</u>-a-peen)

(Seroquel)

Side Effects

Drowsiness
Tardive dyskinesia
Dizziness

Constipation
Hypersensitivity
NMS

Hyperglycemia
Dysphagia
Priapism

Nursing Considerations

- Treatment of schizophrenia and bipolar I disorder, autistic disorder
- Avoid use with alcohol, CNS depressants
- Use caution in potentially hazardous activities
- Avoid changing positions (lying/sitting/standing) rapidly
- Notify clinician if fever, sore throat, bruising/bleeding, tics/spasms, trembling, shuffling gait
- Avoid strenuous exercise in hot weather
- Check before taking OTC meds
- Monitor blood sugar in diabetic patients
- Rx; Preg Cat C

• •

Side Effects

Drowsiness
Dizziness
Hyperglycemia

Hypertension
Dry mouth
Somnolence

Dyspepsia
Weight gain

Nursing Considerations

- Used in treatment of schizophrenia, bipolar I disorder
- Avoid use with alcohol, CNS depressants
- Use caution in potentially hazardous activities
- Avoid changing positions (lying/sitting/standing) rapidly
- Notify clinician if fever, sore throat, bruising/bleeding, tics/spasms, trembling, shuffling gait
- Avoid strenuous exercise in hot weather
- Check before taking OTC meds
- Monitor blood sugar in diabetic patients
- May increase the risk of suicidal thoughts or behavior
- Monitor BP
- May increase ALT
- Rx; Preg Cat C

ZIPRASIDONE HCL
(zye-praz-i-doan)

(Geodon)

• •

Mental Health Medications
Attention Deficit Disorder Agents

METHYLPHENIDATE HCL
(meth-ill-fen-uh-date)

(Concerta, Ritalin)

Side Effects

Drowsiness	Somnolence	Hyperglycemia
Tardive dyskinesia	Abnormal vision	NMS
Dizziness	Vomiting	
Constipation	Headache	

Nursing Considerations

- Used in treatment of schizophrenia, bipolar I disorder
- Avoid use with alcohol, CNS depressants
- Use caution in potentially hazardous activities
- Avoid changing positions (lying/sitting/standing) rapidly
- Notify clinician if fever, sore throat, bruising/bleeding, tics/spasms, trembling, shuffling gait
- Avoid strenuous exercise in hot weather
- Check before taking OTC meds
- Women: avoid breastfeeding
- Monitor blood sugar in diabetic patients
- Rx; Preg Cat C

• •

Side Effects

Headache	Decreased appetite	Nausea
Respiratory infections	Visual disturbance	Insomnia
	Abdominal pain	Restlessness
Hyperhidrosis	Cough	

Nursing Considerations

- Used to treat ADD/ADHD in children over 6 years old and depression in elderly, narcolepsy
- Concerta is time-released and should be swallowed whole, not chewed
- This prescription cannot be refilled
- Dosage is adjusted in 18-mg increments to a maximum of 54 mg/day
- Contraindicated in patients with anxiety, tension, and glaucoma
- This medication may be habit-forming
- May lower seizure threshold
- Monitor for adverse psychiatric symptoms
- Rx; C-II, Preg Cat C

CARBAMAZEPINE
(kar-ba-<u>maz</u>-e-peen)

(Tegretol, Tegretol XR)

· ·

DIVALPROEX SODIUM
(dye-<u>val</u>-proe-ex)

(Depakote)

Side Effects

Myelosuppression	Ataxia	Photosensitivity
Dizziness, drowsiness	Diplopia, rash	Nausea, vomiting

Nursing Considerations

- Management of bipolar disorder, seizures, trigeminal neuralgia, diabetic neuropathy
- Avoid driving and other activities requiring alertness for the first 3 days
- Monitor blood levels, CBC regularly, especially during first 2 months; periodic eye exams
- Take with food or milk to decrease GI upset; tablets (nonextended-release) may be crushed, extended-release capsules may be opened, mixed with juice or soft food
- Urine may turn pink to brown
- Avoid abrupt withdrawal; discontinue gradually
- Avoid use with alcohol, CNS depressants
- Monitor for hepatic reactions
- Monitor thyroid function
- Monitor for suicidal thoughts or behavior
- Patient should wear medical information tag
- Rx; Preg Cat D

• •

Side Effects

Sedation, drowsiness, dizziness	Prolonged bleeding time
Mental status and behavioral changes	Teratogenicity
	Pancreatitis
Nausea, vomiting, constipation, diarrhea, heartburn	Hepatotoxicity

Nursing Considerations

- Management of seizures, manic episodes assoc. with bipolar disorder (delayed-release only), migraine prophylaxis (delayed- and extended-release only)
- Take with or immediately after meals to lessen GI upset
- Swallow tablets or capsules whole (no crushing, chewing)
- Avoid abrupt withdrawal after long-term use; discontinue gradually to prevent convulsions
- Monitor blood levels, platelets, bleeding time, and liver function tests
- Delayed-release products: peak blood level 3–5 hours, duration 12–24 hours
- Extended-release products: peak blood level 7–14 hours, duration 24 hours
- Monitor for suicidal thoughts or behavior
- Wear medical information tag
- Rx; Preg Cat D

LITHIUM
(<u>li</u>-thee-um)

(Lithobid)

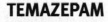

TEMAZEPAM
(tem-<u>az</u>-eh-pam)

(Restoril)

Side Effects

Dizziness
Impaired vision
Fine hand tremors
Reversible leukocytosis

Signs of intoxication:
 vomiting, diarrhea, drowsiness,
 muscular weakness, ataxia

Nursing Considerations

- Controls manic episodes in manic-depressive individuals; mood stabilizer
- Use caution in potentially hazardous activities
- Check serum levels 2 times weekly during treatment, q 2–3 months on maintenance; draw blood in A.M. prior to dose
- Target serum levels: treatment = 0.5 to 1.5 mEq/L, maintenance = 0.6–1.2 mEq/L
- GI symptoms reduced if taken with meals
- Onset of therapeutic effects in 1–2 weeks
- Diabetics: closely monitor blood/urine glucose
- Dose reduced during depressive stages of illness
- Encourage 10–12 glasses water/day and adequate salt intake (6–10 g/day)
- Avoid caffeine, increased exercise, saunas
- Rx; Preg Cat D

• •

Side Effects

Drowsiness
Dizziness
Lethargy
Weakness

Euphoria
Anorexia
Headache
Fatigue

Nursing Considerations

- Used for short-term (7–10 days) treatment of insomnia
- Should be avoided in patients under the age of 18
- Avoid alcohol while taking this drug
- Not intended for use for more than 10 days
- When used with CNS depressants, the CNS depression is increased
- "Sleep driving" may occur, especially if taken with alcohol or CNS depressants
- Rx; C-IV; Preg Cat X

ZALEPLON
(<u>zahl</u>-eh-plahn)

(Sonata)

• •

ZOLPIDEM TARTRATE
(<u>zol</u>-puh-dim)

(Ambien)

Side Effects

Headache

Myalgia

Dizziness

Asthenia

Dyspepsia

Eye pain

Nursing Considerations

- Used in short-term insomnia treatment
- Zaleplon does not prolong sleep time or decrease awakenings
- Elderly patients generally benefit the most
- Because of rapid onset, patients should take immediately before bedtime
- Avoid alcohol while using this medication
- May be habit-forming
- "Sleep driving" may occur
- Rx; C-IV; Preg Cat C

• •

Side Effects

Headache

Drowsiness

Influenza-like symptoms

Dizziness

Nausea

"Drugged" feeling

Nursing Considerations

- Short-term treatment of insomnia
- Dosage may need to be adjusted down if patient is using a CNS depressant to avoid an addictive effect
- Side effects increase with prolonged usage
- May cause "sleep driving"
- May worsen depression
- Monitor for suicidal thoughts or behavior
- Rx; Preg Cat B

ALLOPURINOL
(al-oh-<u>pure</u>-i-nole)

(Aloprim, Zyloprim)

• •

COLCHICINE
(<u>kol</u>-chi-seen)

(Colcrys)

Side Effects

GI upset   Rash
Headache, drowsiness

Nursing Considerations

- Treatment of gout, uric acid neuropathy, uric acid stone formation
- Encourage 10–12 glasses water/day
- Check CBC and renal function tests
- Take with food; don't take vitamin C or iron
- Initial therapy can increase attacks of gout
- Avoid use of alcohol, eating organ meats, gravy, legumes
- Full therapeutic effect may require several months
- Management of patients with leukemia, lymphoma who are receiving chemotherapy that may increase uric acid
- Monitor liver function tests
- Rx; Preg Cat C

• •

Side Effects

Nausea, vomiting, diarrhea   Agranulocytosis
Sign of toxicity: abdominal   Pharyngolaryngeal pain
  cramp

Nursing Considerations

- Treatment and prevention of acute gout attacks, familial Mediterranean fever
- Has analgesic, anti-inflammatory effects
- May be taken without regard to meals
- IV: slowly; do not administer IM/subQ
- Encourage 10–12 glasses water/day
- Avoid use of alcohol, eating organ meats, gravy, legumes
- Always carry medication to treat acute attacks
- Grapefruit and grapefruit juice should not be consumed
- Rx; Preg Cat C

PROBENECID
(proe-<u>ben</u>-e-sid)

(Probalan)

• •

Musculoskeletal Medications
Nonsalicylate NSAIDs, Antirheumatics

DICLOFENAC NA
(dye-<u>kloe</u>-fen-ak)

(Voltaren)

Side Effects

Nausea
Sore gums, anorexia
Hypersensitivity

Skin rash
Hemolytic anemia

Nursing Considerations

- Treatment of hyperuricemia associated with gout, gouty arthritis
- Check BUN, renal function tests
- Encourage 8–10 glasses water/day
- Give with milk, food, and antacids
- Avoid use of alcohol, eating organ meats, gravy, legumes
- May also be used with penicillin to elevate and prolong plasma of penicillin for gonococcal infection
- Avoid aspirin-containing products; may take acetaminophen
- Rx; Preg Cat B

• •

Side Effects

Dizziness
Blood dyscrasias
Headache
Nephrotoxicity

Hypersensitivity
GI distress, bleeding,
  or ulcer
Rash

Nursing Considerations

- Used in arthritic conditions, dysmenorrhea
- Ophthalmic: reduce inflammation after cataract extraction
- PO: take with full glass of water and food and remain upright for 30 minutes
- If dose missed, take within 2 hours
- Use sunscreen to prevent photosensitivity
- May increase risk of cardiovascular thrombotic events
- Possible cross-allergy with aspirin and other NSAIDs
- May increase risk of elevated liver tests
- Rx; Preg Cat C

ETODOLAC
(ee-<u>toe</u>-doe-lak)

• •

Musculoskeletal Medications
Nonsalicylate NSAIDs, Antirheumatics

IBUPROFEN
(eye-byoo-<u>proe</u>-fen)

(Advil, Motrin IB)

Side Effects

Nephrotoxicity

Nausea

Blood dyscrasias

Anorexia

Dizziness

Hypertension

Hypersensitivity

Nursing Considerations

- Reduces pain of osteoarthritis, rheumatoid arthritis
- Monitor for signs of toxicity: blurred vision, ringing or roaring in ears
- Full therapeutic effect may take up to 1 month
- Avoid concurrent use of ASA, NSAIDs, acetaminophen, alcohol
- May increase risk of cardiovascular thrombotic events
- May increase risk of GI bleeding or ulcer
- May cause false positive for urinary bilirubin
- May cause false positive for ketones in urine
- Rx; Preg Cat C

• •

Side Effects

Nausea, vomiting, diarrhea, constipation

Headache, dizziness

Fluid retention

GI bleeding

Hives

Rash

Nursing Considerations

- Treatment of rheumatoid arthritis/osteoarthritis; relief of mild/moderate pain; antipyretic
- Take with milk or food
- Use cautiously with aspirin allergy
- Monitor for visual disturbances, tinnitus
- Monitor for increased weight gain, edema, fever, hematuria, arthralgia
- Avoid alcohol
- OTC, Rx; Preg Cat C

INDOMETHACIN
(in-doe-<u>meth</u>-a-sin)

(Indocin)

• •

NAPROXEN NA
(na-<u>prox</u>-en)

(Aleve, Anaprox, Naprosyn)

Side Effects

Peptic ulcer

Dizziness

Bone marrow depression

Hypersensitivity

Blurred vision

Tinnitus

Hypertension

Drowsiness

Nursing Considerations

- Treatment of rheumatoid arthritis/osteoarthritis, acute gout, acute painful shoulder
- Observe for bleeding problems
- PO: take with food/milk, encourage upright position for 15–30 minutes
- Use caution with potentially hazardous activities
- Avoid use with alcohol, aspirin, other NSAIDs
- May increase risk for cardiovascular thrombotic events
- Monitor for weight gain
- Rx; Preg Cat C

• •

Side Effects

Nausea

Dizziness

Headache

Asthma

GI bleeding

Hives

Nursing Considerations

- For mild to moderate pain; treatment of arthritis, primary dysmenorrhea
- PO: with food to decrease GI upset; on empty stomach to increase absorption
- Monitor for signs of toxicity: blurred vision, ringing or roaring in ears
- Full therapeutic effect may take up to 1 month
- Avoid concurrent use of ASA, steroids, alcohol
- Monitor for melena, weight gain, arthralgia, hematuria
- OTC, Rx; Preg Cat C

PIROXICAM
(peer-<u>ox</u>-i-kam)

(Feldene)

• •

SALSALATE
(<u>sal</u>-sah-late)

(Disalcid)

Side Effects

Drowsiness
Headache
Hypertension

Hypersensitivity
GI disturbances, bleeding
  or ulcer

Nursing Considerations

- For mild to moderate pain, osteoarthritis, rheumatoid arthritis
- PO: with food to decrease GI upset; on empty stomach to increase absorption
- Take at same time every day
- Monitor for signs of toxicity: blurred vision, ringing or roaring in ears, jaundice
- Full therapeutic effect may take up to 1 month
- Avoid concurrent use of ASA, OTC meds, alcohol
- May increase risk of cardiovascular thrombotic events
- Rx; Preg Cat C

• •

Side Effects

Nausea, vomiting
GI bleeding
Vertigo

Heartburn
Rash
Tinnitus

Nursing Considerations

- For mild to moderate pain, rheumatoid arthritis, and osteoarthritis
- PO: can be crushed or taken whole
- PO: take with food or milk to decrease GI upset
- Full therapeutic effect may take 2 weeks
- Read label on OTC meds, may contain ASA
- Monitor for signs of toxicity: changes in liver, kidney, eye, ear functions
- Rx; Preg Cat C

BACLOFEN
(<u>bak</u>-loe-fen)

(Lioresal)

. . . .

CARISOPRODOL
(kar-eye-soe-<u>proe</u>-dole)

(Soma)

Side Effects

Drowsiness
Dizziness
Weakness, fatigue
Confusion

Nausea, vomiting
Headache
Seizures

Nursing Considerations

- Used to reduce spasticity in multiple sclerosis, spinal cord injury, flexor spasms, and muscular rigidity
- Take with food
- Avoid alcohol, CNS depressants
- Increased risk of seizures in patients with seizure disorder
- Withdraw gradually over 1 to 2 weeks, unless severe adverse reactions; D/C may cause hallucinations, tachycardia, or rebound spasticity
- Monitor for symptoms of sensitivity: fever, skin eruptions, respiratory distress
- May elevate blood sugar, monitor blood sugar in diabetic patients
- Rx; Preg Cat C

• •

Side Effects

Drowsiness
Light-headedness
Headache

Dizziness
Nausea

Nursing Considerations

- Relief of pain, stiffness associated with musculoskeletal conditions
- PO: onset 30 minutes, peak 4 hours, duration 4–6 hours
- Avoid alcohol, CNS depressants, including OTC cold or allergy meds
- Avoid activities requiring alertness until effects of medication are known
- May cause dependence; this is not a controlled substance
- Rx; Preg Cat C

CYCLOBENZAPRINE
(sye-kole-<u>ben</u>-za-preen)

(Flexeril)

. . . .

METAXALONE
(meh-<u>tax</u>-uh-lone)

(Skelaxin)

Side Effects

Drowsiness

Dizziness

Fatigue

Dry mouth

Constipation

Headache

Nursing Considerations

- Relieves muscle spasms from acute conditions
- Avoid alcohol, CNS depressants, including OTC cold or allergy meds
- Avoid activities requiring alertness until effects of medication are known
- Rx; Preg Cat B

• •

Side Effects

Drowsiness

Gastrointestinal pains

Nervousness

Dizziness

Headache

Irritability

Nursing Considerations

- Used to relieve painful musculoskeletal injuries
- Should be an adjunct to rest and physical therapy
- Avoid alcohol while using this drug
- Use caution when operating machinery
- Use cautiously in patients with known liver impairment
- May cause false positive Benedict's test
- Rx; Preg Cat N/A

METHOCARBAMOL
(meth-oh-<u>kar</u>-ba-mole)

(Robaxin)

. . . .

Neurological Medications
Neurological Medications

BENZTROPINE
(<u>benz</u>-troe-peen)

(Cogentin)

Side Effects

Drowsiness	Dizziness
Light-headedness	Nausea

Nursing Considerations

- Relieves muscle spasms from acute conditions, tetanus management
- IM: inject deep into UOQ of buttock, rotate sites
- NG tube: crush tablets into fluid
- PO: take with food or milk
- Metallic taste may develop
- Urine may turn green, black, or brown
- Avoid alcohol, CNS depressants, including OTC cold or allergy meds
- Avoid activities requiring alertness until effects of medication are known
- Monitor IV sites carefully for extravasation
- Rx; Preg Cat C

• •

Side Effects

Dry mouth	Weakness
Constipation	Tardive dyskinesia
Anhidrosis	

Nursing Considerations

- Treatment of Parkinson symptoms, EPS associated with neuroleptic drugs, acute dystonic reactions
- IM/IV: onset 15 minutes, duration 6–10 hours
- PO: onset 1 hour, duration 6–10 hours
- Tablets may be crushed and mixed with food
- Taper med over a week, or withdrawal symptoms: EPS, tremors, insomnia, tachycardia, restlessness
- Avoid hazardous activities until stabilized on med
- Change positions slowly
- Avoid alcohol, antihistamines unless directed by clinician
- Antidote is physostigmine
- Rx; Preg Cat C

CAFFEINE/ERGOTAMINE
(er-<u>got</u>-a-meen)

(Cafergot)

· ·

CARBIDOPA/LEVODOPA
(kar-bih-<u>doe</u>-pa/<u>leev</u>-oe-doe-pa)

(Sinemet)

Side Effects

Headache

Tremors, convulsions

Blood vessel contraction,
  with decreased circulation,
  esp. in limbs

Toxic erotism: nausea, vomiting,
  diarrhea, dizziness, headache,
  mental confusion

Nursing Considerations

- Treatment of vascular headache
- Take at onset of pain/during prodromal stage to abort headache
- Lie down in darkened quiet room for several hours
- Rx; Preg Cat X

• •

Side Effects

Twitching

Headache, dizziness

Mental changes: confusion,
  agitation, mood alterations

Dark urine/sweat

Cardiac arrhythmias

Nursing Considerations

- Treatment for Parkinson disease and syndrome
- Replacement dopaminergic agent
- Change positions slowly
- Take with food; decreased effect with liver, pork, wheat germ,
  and vitamin B6
- Full therapeutic effect may take several months
- Monitor for melanoma
- May cause dark color in saliva, urine, or sweat
- May increase liver function test results
- May cause false positive for urine ketones
- Rx; Preg Cat C

DONEPEZIL
(doe-<u>nep</u>-uh-zill)

(Aricept)

· ·

ELETRIPTAN HYDROBROMIDE
(e-le-<u>trip</u>-tan hi-dro-<u>bro</u>-mide)

(Relpax)

Side Effects

Nausea, vomiting, diarrhea
Headache, dizziness
Fatigue
Twitching
Cardiac arrhythmias
Insomnia

Seizures
Rash
Dark urine/sweat
Mental changes: confusion,
  agitation, mood alterations

Nursing Considerations

- Used in treatment of mild to moderate Alzheimer's disease
- Drug does not cure, but stabilizes or relieves symptoms
- Take at regular intervals
- Take between meals or may be given with meals to decrease GI upset
- May increase BUN, SGOT, GPT
- Rx; Preg Cat C

• •

Side Effects

Coronary artery vasospasm
Transient myocardial ischemia
MI
Ventricular tachycardia
Ventricular fibrillation
Asthenia

Nausea
Dizziness
Somnolence
Hypertension
Diaphoresis
Seizure

Nursing Considerations

- Indicated for treatment of migraine headaches with and without aura
- May be taken with or without food
- Teach patient to call physician or seek immediate medical help for chest pain or SOB
- Teach patient to call physician or seek immediate medical help for confusion, hallucinations, tachycardia, feeling faint, fever, diaphoresis, muscle spasm, or difficulty walking
- Rx; Preg Cat C

METHYLPHENIDATE
(meth-ill-<u>fen</u>-i-date)

(Concerta, Ritalin)

• •

SELEGILINE
(se-<u>le</u>-ji-leen)

(Eldepryl)

Side Effects

Hyperactivity, insomnia	Palpitations, tachycardia	Visual disturbance
Restlessness	Hyperhidrosis	Nausea
Talkativeness	Anorexia	Abdominal pain
		Cough

Nursing Considerations

- Management of attention deficit hyperactive disorder, narcolepsy, depression in the elderly
- Onset 30 minutes, duration 4–6 hours
- Take at least 6 hours before bedtime (regular-release) or 10 hours before bedtime (sustained-release, extended-release)
- Taper med over several weeks or depression, increased sleeping, lethargy will occur
- Avoid hazardous activities until stabilized on med
- Decrease caffeine consumption (coffee, tea, cola, chocolate) to decrease irritability
- Monitor for adverse psychiatric symptoms
- May lower seizure threshold
- Rx; C-II; Preg Cat C

• •

Side Effects

Dizziness	Nausea	Dyspepsia
Cardiac dysrhythmias	Pain	Insomnia
Rhinitis	Headache	
	Back pain	

Nursing Considerations

- Indirect-acting dopaminergic agent
- Used in management of Parkinson disease with levodopa/carbidopa
- Do not use with tricyclics or opioids; do not use with meperidine
- Monitor for signs of toxicity: twitching, eye spasms
- Do not stop abruptly; parkinsonian crisis may occur
- Avoid foods high in tyramine: cheese, pickled products, alcohol, large amounts of caffeine
- Monitor for melanoma
- Monitor for intense urges (gambling, sexual)
- Rx; Preg Cat C

ZOLMITRIPTAN
(zole-mih-<u>trip</u>-tan)

(Zomig)

• •

DORZOLAMIDE HCL
(dor-<u>zoh</u>-la-mide)

(Trusopt)

Side Effects

Weakness, neck stiffness

Tingling, hot sensation,
  burning, feeling of pressure,
  tightness

Numbness, dizziness, sedation

Hypertension

Dyspepsia

Dry mouth

Nursing Considerations

- Used for treatment of acute migraine with or without aura
- Take as soon as symptoms occur
- PO: tablet may be split
- Avoid foods high in tyramine: cheese, pickled products, alcohol, large amounts of caffeine
- May cause serotonin syndrome when used with antidepression medication
- Rx; Preg Cat C

• •

Side Effects

Ocular burning, stinging,
  discomfort

Blurred vision, tearing,
  or dryness

Photophobia

Bitter taste in mouth

Nursing Considerations

- Treatment of glaucoma and ocular hypertension
- Wash hands before and after instillation
- Do not touch tip of dropper to eye or body
- Do not wear contact lens during instillation
- Drug is a sulfonamide; although given topically, it can be absorbed systemically
- Stop if eye inflammation or eyelid reactions
- Rx; Preg Cat C

DORZOLAMIDE/TIMOLOL
(dor-<u>zoh</u>-la-mide/<u>tye</u>-moe-lole)

(Cosopt)

• •

TRAVOPROST
(<u>trav</u>-oh-prahst)

(Travatan)

Side Effects

Ocular burning, stinging, discomfort
Blurred vision, tearing, or dryness

Photophobia
Bitter taste in mouth

Nursing Considerations

- Treatment of glaucoma and ocular hypertension
- Place pressure on tear ducts for 1 minute
- Wash hands before and after instillation
- Do not touch drug container to eye or body
- Do not wear contact lens during instillation
- Drug contains sulfonamide; although given topically, it can be absorbed systemically
- Stop if eye inflammation or eyelid reactions
- Rx; Preg Cat C

. . . .

Side Effects

Ocular hyperemia
Decreased visual acuity
Eye discomfort or pain

Foreign-body sensation
Eye pruritus

Nursing Considerations

- Treatment of glaucoma and ocular hypertension for patients who can't tolerate or respond inadequately to other IOP-lowering drugs
- Place pressure on tear ducts for 1 minute
- Wash hands before and after instillation
- Do not touch tip of dropper to eye or body
- Potential for increased brown pigmentation of iris, eyelid skin darkening, changes in eyelashes; important if only one eye is being treated
- Stop if eye inflammation or eyelid reactions
- Remove contact lens to give med; can reinsert in 15 minutes
- Discard med 6 months after opening
- Rx; Preg Cat C

LEVOBUNOLOL
(lee-voe-<u>byoo</u>-no-lole)

(AK-Beta, Betagan)

• •

TIMOLOL
(<u>tim</u>-oh-lole)

(Timoptic, Betimol solution)

Side Effects

Hypotension

Transient eye stinging
and burning

Asthma attacks in patients
with history of asthma

Bradycardia

Nursing Considerations

- Treatment of glaucoma and ocular hypertension
- Place pressure on tear ducts for 1 minute
- Wash hands before and after instillation
- Do not touch tip of dropper to eye or body
- Drug is a beta blocker
- Although given topically, it can be absorbed systemically
- Report shortness of breath, chest pain, or heart irregularity
- Monitor diabetic patients for hypoglycemia
- Wear medical information tag
- Rx; Preg Cat C

• •

Side Effects

Fatigue

Weakness

Hypotension

Burning and stinging
of eye

Bradycardia

Nursing Considerations

- Treatment of glaucoma and ocular hypertension
- Place pressure on tear ducts for 1 minute
- Wash hands before and after instillation
- Do not touch drug container to eye or body
- Monitor for hypoglycemia in diabetic patients
- Rx; Preg Cat C

BRIMONIDINE TARTRATE
(brih-<u>moh</u>-nih-deen)

(Alphagan P)

• •

CROMOLYN NA
(<u>kroe</u>-moe-lin)

(Opticrom)

Side Effects

Ocular hyperemia
Allergic conjunctivitis
Pruritus

Fatigue
Hypertension
Visual disturbance

Nursing Considerations

- Treatment of glaucoma and ocular hypertension
- Wait 15 minutes after use to wear soft contact lens
- Use caution with hazardous activities due to decreased
  mental alertness
- Avoid alcohol
- Monitor intraocular pressure because may reverse after
  1 month of therapy
- Rx; Preg Cat B

• •

Side Effects

Ocular irritation
Hypersensitivity

Nursing Considerations

- Used in treatment of conjunctivitis, keratitis
- Wash hands before and after instillation
- Do not touch tip of dropper to eye or body
- Do not wear soft contact lens while using this medication
- Rx; Preg Cat B

FLURBIPROFEN
(flur-bi-<u>proe</u>-fen)

(Ocufen)

• •

ANTIPYRINE/BENZOCAINE/ GLYCERIN OTIC SOLUTION
(Auralgan)

Side Effects
Ocular irritation

Nursing Considerations
- Inhibition of intraoperative miosis
- Give every 30 minutes, starting 2 hours before surgery, 4 drops to each eye
- May cause increase bleed of ocular tissue with ocular surgery
- Rx; Preg Cat C

• •

Side Effects
Hypersensitivity

Nursing Considerations
- Otic analgesic inflammation
- Suspension: shake well (also comes in solution)
- Can warm up with hands for patient's comfort
- Warn patient not to touch ear with dropper
- Warn patient that drug is for use in ears only
- Do not get in eyes, nose, or mouth
- May place cotton plug moistened with Auralgan in ear canal
- Do not rinse dropper
- Rx; Preg Cat N/A

HYDROCORTISONE/NEOMYCIN/ POLYMYXIN OTIC

(Cortisporin)

· ·

ALBUTEROL/ IPRATROPIUM INHALER

(al-byoo-tear-ol/eye-pra-troe-pee-um)

(Combivent)

Side Effects

Hypersensitivity
Burning

Dryness
Skin atrophy

Nursing Considerations

- Otic analgesic and antibiotic for treatment of bacterial infections of external auditory canal
- Warn patient not to touch ear with dropper
- Explain drug is for use in ears only
- Possible cross allergy with kanamycin, paromomycin, streptomycin, and gentamicin
- Rx; Preg Cat C

● ●

Side Effects

Nervousness, hyperactivity, tremors
Dry mouth, photophobia, constipation
Tachycardia, palpitations
Nausea, vomiting

Headache
URI
Dyspnea
Cough
Bronchitis
Hypersensitivity

Nursing Considerations

- Treatment of COPD
- Teach how to correctly use inhaler
- Monitor for toxicity
- Assess for hypersensitivity, including soy products, atropine, peanuts
- Encourage 10–12 glasses water/day
- Avoid OTC cough/hay-fever medications
- Use caution with hazardous activities
- Rx; Preg Cat C

CROMOLYN SODIUM INHALER
(<u>kroe</u>-moe-lin)

(Intal)

• •

MONTELUKAST
(mon-tea-<u>lew</u>-cast)

(Singulair)

Side Effects

Bronchospasm
Cough, wheeze

Dizziness
Nausea

Nursing Considerations

- Prophylactic management of bronchial asthma
- Notify clinician of wheezing, respiratory distress
- Do not use for acute asthma attacks
- Full therapeutic effect may take several weeks
- Rx; Preg Cat B

• •

Side Effects

Dizziness
Headache
URI
Fever

Pharyngitis
Cough
GI upset
Otitis media

Runny nose
Sinusitis

Nursing Considerations

- Prophylaxis and treatment of chronic asthma and allergic rhinitis
- Do not use to treat acute symptoms; use a rapid-acting bronchodilator
- Notify clinician of wheezing, respiratory distress
- Full therapeutic effect may take several weeks
- May increase risk of neuropsychiatric events including hallucination, aggression, anxiousness, suicidal behavior and thinking, and tremor
- Rx; Preg Cat B

THEOPHYLLINE
(thee-<u>off</u>-i-lin)

. . . .

BENZONATATE
(ben-<u>zoe</u>-na-tate)

(Tessalon)

Side Effects

Restlessness	Dizziness	Headache
Palpitations, sinus tachycardia	Anorexia Vomiting	Insomnia

Nursing Considerations

- Treatment of bronchial asthma, bronchospasm of COPD, chronic bronchitis, emphysema
- PO: peak 2 hours; take with full glass of water; best on empty stomach
- Solution: peak 1 hour
- Check all OTC and other meds for ephedrine before taking with this med
- Avoid alcohol, caffeine, smoking
- Avoid activities requiring alertness until response to med is known
- Contact clinician if toxicity: nausea, vomiting, anxiety, insomnia, convulsions
- Drink 8–10 glasses of fluid per day
- Do not crush enteric-coated SR preparations, swallow whole
- Rx; Preg Cat C

• •

Side Effects

Dizziness	Sedation headache
Drowsiness	Nausea
Rash	

Nursing Considerations

- Treatment of nonproductive cough
- PO: onset 15–20 minutes, duration 3–8 hours
- Capsules should be swallowed whole; do not chew, because release of med may cause local anesthetic effect and choking
- Additive CNS depression may occur with antihistamines, alcohol, opioids, and sedative/hypnotics
- Avoid activities requiring alertness until response to med is known
- Contact clinician if signs of overdose: convulsions, trembling, restlessness
- Check lungs regularly
- Rx; Preg Cat C

HYDROCODONE
(hye-droe-<u>koe</u>-done)

(Hycodan; with acetaminophen, Vicodin)

• •

IPRATROPIUM BROMIDE
(eye-pra-<u>troe</u>-pee-um)

(Atrovent)

Side Effects

Nausea, vomiting
Anorexia
Circulatory and
  respiratory depression

Constipation
Drowsiness

Nursing Considerations

- Treatment of hyperactive and nonproductive cough, mild pain relief
- Physical dependency may result when used for extended periods
- Withdrawal symptoms may occur: nausea, vomiting, cramps, fever, faintness, anorexia
- Avoid CNS depressants
- Onset: 10–20 minutes, duration 4–6 hours
- Do not perform potentially dangerous tasks after taking medication
- Rx; Preg Cat C-III

• •

Side Effects

Nervousness
Tremors
Dry mouth
Palpitations
URI

Epistaxis (nosebleed)
Rhinitis
Pharyngitis
Angioedema

Nursing Considerations

- Treatment of bronchospasm associated with COPD, rhinorrhea, rhinitis
- Not for acute bronchospasm needing rapid response
- Teach use of metered dose inhaler: inhale, hold breath, exhale slowly
- Don't mix in nebulizer with cromolyn sodium
- Assess for hypersensitivity, including soy products, atropine, peanuts
- Encourage 10–12 glasses water/day
- Avoid OTC cough/hayfever medications
- Use caution with hazardous activities
- Rx; Preg Cat B

ALBUTEROL SULFATE
(al-<u>byoo</u>-tear-ol)

(Proventil-HFA, ProAir HFA)

• •

SALMETEROL
(sal-<u>me</u>-teh-role)

(Serevent)

Side Effects

Tremors
Headache
Hyperactivity
Tachycardia
Nausea, vomiting

URI
Rhinitis
Hypersensitivity
GI upset

Nursing Considerations

- Treatment of bronchial asthma, reversible bronchospasm, prevention of exercise-induced asthma
- Teach patient how to correctly use inhaler
- Monitor for toxicity
- PO: take with food to decrease GI upset; may crush tablets
- Teach patient how to take radial pulse
- Rx; Preg Cat C

. . . .

Side Effects

Headache
Hypersensitivity
URI

Throat irritation
Myalgia
Nausea, vomiting

Nursing Considerations

- Long-term control of asthma, prevention of exercise-induced asthma, prevention of bronchospasm in COPD
- Do not use to treat acute symptoms; do not as a use a rapid-acting bronchodilator
- Contact clinician if difficulty breathing, if more inhalations are needed of rapid-acting bronchodilator, using more than four inhalations of a rapid-acting bronchodilator for 2 or more consecutive days, or more than one canister in 8 weeks
- Teach patient inhaler setup and use
- Avoid exposure to chickenpox and measles
- Rx; Preg Cat C

TERBUTALINE SULFATE
(ter-<u>byoo</u>-ta-leen)

· ·

GUAIFENESIN
(gwye-<u>fen</u>-e-sin)

(Robitussin, Mucinex, Mytussin)

Side Effects

Nervousness

Restlessness

Tremor

Palpations

Chest pains

Rapid pulse

Headache

Nursing Considerations

- Management of asthma or COPD and bronchospasm
- Inhalation and subQ used for short-term control; PO as long-term
- PO: take with food to decrease GI upset
- Tablets may be crushed and mixed with food or fluids
- subQ: give injections in lateral deltoid
- Contact clinician if unrelieved shortness of breath
- Teach patient how to take radial pulse
- Rx; Preg Cat B

• •

Side Effects

Nausea

Nursing Considerations

- Helps loosen mucous and bronchial secretions to make coughs more productive
- PO: onset 30 minutes, duration 4–6 hours
- PO extended-release: duration 12 hours
- Do not crush pills
- Take with full glass of water
- OTC, Rx; Preg Cat C

CROMOLYN SODIUM
(<u>kroe</u>-moe-lin)

(NasalCrom)

• •

DISULFIRAM
(dye-<u>sul</u>-fih-ram)

(Antabuse)

Side Effects

Nasal burning and irritation
Headache
Bad taste

Epistaxis (nosebleed)
Postnasal drip

Nursing Considerations

- Prophylaxis and treatment of allergic rhinitis
- Full therapeutic effect may take several weeks
- Rx; Preg Cat B

• •

Side Effects

In the absence of alcohol: drowsiness, headache, restlessness, fatigue
In the presence of alcohol: flushing, chest pain, heart arrhythmias,
  hypotension, seizures, throbbing in head and neck, sweating

Nursing Considerations

- Used for treatment of chronic alcoholism by causing severe
  hypersensitivity
- Onset may be delayed up to 12 hours; single dose may be effective
  for 1–2 weeks
- Never give without patient's knowledge
- Avoid alcohol in any form: in foods, sauces, or other meds, such
  as cough syrups or tonics
- Avoid vinegar, paregoric, skin products, liniments, or lotions
  containing alcohol
- Do not begin treatment for at least 12 hours after drinking alcohol
- Wear medical information tag
- Rx; Preg Cat C

CARBONYL IRON

• •

FERRIC GLUCONATE COMPLEX
(Ferrlecit)

Side Effects

Nausea, constipation
Epigastric pain

Black and red tarry stools

Nursing Considerations

- Treatment of iron deficiency anemia, prophylaxis for iron deficiency in pregnancy
- Contains 100% elemental iron
- Keep upright for 15–30 minutes to avoid esophageal corrosion, take 1 hour before bedtime
- Stools will become black or dark green
- Do not substitute one iron salt for another because iron content differs
- Do not take within 1 hour before or 2 hours after antacids, eggs, whole-grain bread or cereal, milk, coffee, or tea
- Rx; Preg Cat A

• •

Side Effects

Nausea, constipation
Epigastric pain
Black and red tarry stools
Hypersensitivity
Injection site reaction

Chest pain
Fatigue
Cramps
Hypotension
Itching

Nursing Considerations

- Treatment of iron deficiency anemia in dialysis patients, given IV
- Onset 4 days, peak 1–2 weeks
- Stools will become black or dark green
- Do not mix with other medication
- Only mix with 0.9% sodium chloride
- Rx; Preg Cat B

FERROUS FUMARATE

(Femiron, Feostat)

· ·

FERROUS GLUCONATE

(Fergon)

Side Effects

Nausea, constipation   Black and red tarry stools
Epigastric pain

Nursing Considerations

- Treatment of iron deficiency anemia, prophylaxis for iron deficiency in pregnancy
- Contains 33% elemental iron
- Keep upright for 15–30 minutes to avoid esophageal corrosion; take 1 hour before bedtime
- Stools will become black or dark green
- Do not substitute one iron salt for another because iron content differs
- Give 1 hour before or 2 hours after meals
- Liquid may stain teeth
- Do not take within 1 hour before or 2 hours after antacids, eggs, whole-grain bread or cereal, milk, coffee, or tea
- Rx; Preg Cat A

• •

Side Effects

Nausea, constipation   Black and red tarry stools
Epigastric pain

Nursing Considerations

- Treatment of iron deficiency anemia, prophylaxis for iron deficiency in pregnancy
- Contains 12% elemental iron
- Keep upright for 15–30 minutes to avoid esophageal corrosion; take 1 hour before bedtime
- Stools will become black or dark green
- Take on empty stomach, if possible
- Do not substitute one iron salt for another because iron content differs
- Liquid may stain teeth
- Do not take 1 hour before or 2 hours after antacids, eggs, whole-grain bread or cereal, milk, coffee, or tea
- Rx; Preg Cat A

FERROUS SULFATE
(Feosol)

• •

IRON POLYSACCHARIDE
(Niferex)

Side Effects

Nausea, constipation
Epigastric pain

Black and red tarry stools

Nursing Considerations

- Treatment of iron deficiency anemia, prophylaxis for iron deficiency in pregnancy
- Contains 30% elemental iron
- Keep upright for 15–30 minutes to avoid esophageal corrosion; take 1 hour before bedtime
- Stools will become black or dark green
- May be taken with or without food
- Do not substitute one iron salt for another because iron content differs
- Liquid may stain teeth
- Do not take within 1 hour or 2 hours after antacids, eggs, whole-grain bread or cereal, milk, coffee, or tea
- Rx; Preg Cat A

• •

Side Effects

Nausea, constipation
Epigastric pain

Black and red tarry stools

Nursing Considerations

- Treatment of iron deficiency anemia, prophylaxis for iron deficiency in pregnancy
- Keep upright for 15–30 minutes to avoid esophageal corrosion; take 1 hour before bedtime
- Stools will become black or dark green
- Take on empty stomach, if possible; may be taken with food
- Do not substitute one iron salt for another because iron content differs
- Liquid may stain teeth
- Do not take within 1 hour or 2 hours after antacids, eggs, whole-grain bread or cereal, milk, coffee, or tea
- Rx; Preg Cat A

Treatment/Replacement
Minerals

POTASSIUM

· ·

Treatment/Replacement
Narcotic Antagonists

NALOXONE HCL
(nal-<u>ox</u>-own)

Side Effects

Nausea, vomiting   Cramps, diarrhea

Nursing Considerations

- Prevention and treatment of hypokalemia
- Onset for PO 30 minutes, IV immediate
- Do not give IM, subQ
- Avoid OTC antacids, salt substitutes, analgesics, vitamins unless directed by clinician
- Report hyperkalemia: lethargy, confusion, GI symptoms, fainting, decreased output
- Report continued hypokalemia: fatigue, weakness, polyuria, polydipsia, cardiac changes
- Do not give IV push
- Do not infuse faster than 10 mg/hr in adults
- Give PO while patient is sitting up or standing
- Dilute liquid prior to giving via NG
- Monitor IV infusions for extravasation; IV infusions may sting or burn
- OTC, Rx; Preg Cat C

• •

Side Effects

Withdrawal symptoms in narcotic-dependent patients: restlessness, muscle spasms, tearing

Nursing Considerations

- Used to reverse narcotic depression, including respiratory symptoms
- IM and subQ onset in 2–5 minutes; IV 1–2 minutes
- Have emergency support equipment available
- May increase PTT
- Monitor for bleeding in surgical and obstetric patients
- Rx; Preg Cat C

ERGOCALCIFEROL
(er-goe-kal-<u>sif</u>-e-role)

(Vitamin D2)

• •

CYANOCOBALAMIN
(sye-an-oh-koe-<u>bal</u>-a-min)

(Vitamin B12)

Side Effects

Metallic taste, dry mouth
Hypervitaminosis D

Nursing Considerations

- Treatment of vitamin D deficiency, rickets, psoriasis, rheumatoid arthritis, hypoparathyroidism
- If med is missed, omit
- Decrease use of antacids and laxatives containing magnesium
- Mineral oil interferes with absorption
- Rx; Preg Cat C

• •

Side Effects

Diarrhea

Nursing Considerations

- Treatment of vitamin B12 deficiency, pernicious anemia, hemorrhage, renal and hepatic disease
- IM, subQ, nasal: peak 3–10 days
- Foods high in this vitamin: meats, seafood, egg yolk, fermented cheeses
- Excessive intake of alcohol or vitamin C may decrease oral absorption/effectiveness
- OTC, Rx; Preg Cat A

FOLIC ACID
(<u>foe</u>-lik <u>a</u>-cid)

· ·

HYDROXOCOBALAMIN
(hye-<u>drox</u>-o-ko-bal-a-min)

(Vitamin B12)

Side Effects
Bronchospasm
Hypersensitivity

Nursing Considerations
- Treatment of anemia, liver disease, alcoholism, intestinal obstruction, pregnancy due to folic acid deficiency
- Also contained in bran, yeast, dried beans, nuts, fruits, fresh vegetables, asparagus
- OTC; Preg Cat A

• •

Side Effects
Diarrhea
Hypersensitivity

Nursing Considerations
- Treatment of vitamin B12 deficiency, pernicious anemia, hemorrhage, renal and hepatic disease
- IM, subQ: peak 3–10 days
- Foods high in this vitamin: meats, seafood, egg yolk, fermented cheeses
- OTC, Rx; Preg Cat A

NIACINAMIDE
(nye-ah-<u>sin</u>-ah-myd)

. . . .

Women's Health
Contraceptives, Systemic

DESOGESTREL/
ETHINYL ESTRADIOL
(dess-oh-<u>jes</u>-trel/<u>eth</u>-in-il es-tra-<u>dye</u>-ole)

(Cyclessa, Desogen, Mircette, Ortho-Cept)

Side Effects

Headache
Nausea

Postural hypotension
Flushing

Nursing Considerations

- Prophylaxis and treatment of pellagra, high cholesterol
- Take with meals to reduce GI upset, can add 325 mg ASA 30 minutes before dose to reduce flushing
- Flushing will occur several hours after med is taken, will decrease over 2 weeks
- Avoid changing positions (sitting/standing/lying) rapidly
- NSAIDs may reduce flushing
- OTC, Rx; Preg Cat C

• •

Side Effects

Headache
Breakthrough bleeding,
  spotting

Contact lens intolerance
Dizziness
Nausea

Nursing Considerations

- Prevention of pregnancy, treatment of endometriosis, hypermenorrhea (monophasic)
- Counsel patient to contact clinician if unusual bleeding, severe headache, difficulty breathing, changes in vision/coordination, chest/leg pain
- Counsel patient this medication does not protect against STDs or HIV
- Avoid smoking, which increases risk of adverse cardiovascular events
- Stop med for at least 1 week before surgery to decrease risk of thromboembolism
- St. John's wort may decrease effectiveness
- Rx; Preg Cat X

DROSPIRENONE/ ETHINYL ESTRADIOL

(dro-<u>spy</u>-re-nown/<u>eth</u>-in-il <u>ess</u>-tra-dy-ol)

(Yaz)

• •

ETHINYL ESTRADIOL/ ETHYNODIOL

(<u>eth</u>-in-il es-tra-<u>dye</u>-ole/e-thye-noe-<u>dye</u>-ole)

(Demulen)

Side Effects

Headache
Breast pain
Vaginal itching,
   discharge, or
   yeast infection
Nausea

Painful menstrual
   period, menstrual
   disorder, break-
   through bleeding
Increase in BP
Sinusitis

Weakness
URI
Weight gain
Symptoms of
   depression
UTI

Nursing Considerations

- Used to prevent pregnancy, as treatment for PMDD and moderate acne vulgaris
- Take at the same time daily, once a day
- Avoid smoking, which increases risk of adverse cardiovascular events
- Counsel patient this medication does not protect against STDs or HIV
- Teach patient to promptly report any visual disturbances, unusual bleeding, chest or leg pain, change in coordination, dyspnea, or severe headache
- Monitor BP
- May increase risk of cardiovascular events including MI and stroke
- St. John's wort may decrease effectiveness
- Rx; Preg Cat X

• •

Side Effects

Headache
Breakthrough bleeding,
   spotting

Dizziness
Nausea
Contact lens intolerance

Nursing Considerations

- Prevention of pregnancy, treatment of endometriosis, hypermenorrhea (monophasic)
- Counsel patient this medication does not protect against STDs or HIV
- Contact clinician if unusual bleeding, severe headache, difficulty breathing, changes in vision/coordination, chest/leg pain
- Avoid smoking, which increases risk of adverse cardiovascular events
- Stop med for at least 1 week before surgery to decrease risk of thromboembolism
- St. John's wort may decrease effectiveness
- Rx; Preg Cat X

ETHINYL ESTRADIOL/ NORETHINDRONE

(<u>eth</u>-in-il es-tra-<u>dye</u>-ole/nor-eth-<u>in</u>-drone)

(Ortho-Novum 1/35)

• •

ETHINYL ESTRADIOL/ NORETHINDRONE

(<u>eth</u>-in-il es-tra-<u>dye</u>-ole/nor-eth-<u>in</u>-drone)

(Ortho-Novum 7-7-7)

Side Effects

Headache

Breakthrough bleeding, spotting

Contact lens intolerance

Dizziness

Nausea

Nursing Considerations

- Prevention of pregnancy, treatment of endometriosis, hypermenorrhea (monophasic)
- Counsel patient this medication does not protect against STDs or HIV
- Contact clinician if unusual bleeding, severe headache, difficulty breathing, changes in vision/coordination, chest/leg pain
- Avoid smoking, which increases risk of adverse cardiovascular events
- Stop med for at least 1 week before surgery to decrease risk of thromboembolism
- St. John's wort may decrease effectiveness
- Rx; Preg Cat X

• •

Side Effects

Nausea

Bloating

Headache

Breakthrough bleeding

Contact lens intolerance

Dizziness

Nursing Considerations

- Female contraception (triphasic)
- Counsel patient this medication does not protect against STDs or HIV
- Contact clinician if breast lumps, vaginal bleeding, edema, jaundice, dark urine, clay-colored stools, dyspnea, headache, blurred vision, abdominal pain, numbness or stiffness in legs, chest pain, tenderness with redness and swelling in extremities
- Contact clinician if weekly weight gain is over 5 pounds
- Can take with food or milk to decrease GI upset
- St. John's wort may decrease effectiveness
- Rx; Preg Cat X

ETHINYL ESTRADIOL/ NORGESTREL
(<u>eth</u>-in-il es-tra-<u>dye</u>-ole/nor-<u>jess</u>-trel)

(Ogestrel, Ovral)

. . . .

LEVONORGESTREL
(lee-voe-nor-<u>jess</u>-trel)

(Mirena)

Side Effects

Headache

Breakthrough bleeding, spotting

Contact lens intolerance

Dizziness

Nausea

Nursing Considerations

- Prevention of pregnancy, treatment of endometriosis, hypermenorrhea (monophasic)
- Counsel patient this medication does not protect against STDs or HIV
- Contact clinician if unusual bleeding, severe headache, difficulty breathing, changes in vision/coordination, chest/leg pain
- Avoid smoking, which increases risk of adverse cardiovascular events
- Stop med for at least 1 week before surgery to decrease risk of thromboembolism
- St. John's wort may decrease effectiveness
- Rx; Preg Cat X

• •

Side Effects

Breakthrough bleeding

Amenorrhea

Ovarian cysts

Abdominal pain

Nursing Considerations

- Prevention of pregnancy for 5 years as a contraceptive implant; emergency contraceptive in oral form
- Implant: onset 1 month, peak 1 month, duration 5 years
- Implant: six capsules are implanted in the upper arm during the first 7 days after onset of menses
- PO for emergency contraceptive: given within 72 hours of unprotected intercourse and repeated 12 hours later
- Available as IUD with medication reservoir
- Counsel patient this medication does not protect against STDs or HIV
- Monitor for PID
- Monitor glucose levels in diabetic patients
- St. John's wort may decrease effectiveness
- Rx; Preg Cat X

MESTRANOL/
NORETHINDRONE

(<u>mes</u>-tre-nole/nor-eth-<u>in</u>-drone)

(Norinyl)

• •

NORETHINDRONE

(nor-eth-<u>in</u>-drone)

(Micronor, Nor-Qd)

Side Effects

Headache

Breakthrough bleeding,
  spotting

Contact lens intolerance

Dizziness

Nausea

Nursing Considerations

- Prevention of pregnancy, treatment of endometriosis, hypermenorrhea (monophasic)
- Counsel patient this medication does not protect against STDs or HIV
- Contact clinician if unusual bleeding, severe headache, difficult breathing, changes in vision/coordination, chest/leg pain
- Avoid smoking, which increases risk of adverse cardiovascular events
- Stop med for at least 1 week before surgery to decrease risk of thromboembolism
- St. John's wort may decrease effectiveness
- Rx; Preg Cat X

• •

Side Effects

Nausea

Headache

Irregular bleeding (genital)

Nursing Considerations

- Management of abnormal uterine bleeding, amenorrhea, endometriosis, contraception
- Counsel patient this medication does not protect against STDs or HIV
- Contact clinician if breast lumps, vaginal bleeding, edema, jaundice, dark urine, clay-colored stools, dyspnea, headache, blurred vision, abdominal pain, numbness or stiffness in legs, chest pain, tenderness with redness and swelling in extremities
- Contact clinician if weekly weight gain is over 5 pounds
- Can take with food or milk to decrease GI upset
- Cigarette smoking increases risk of serious cardiovascular disease
- Rx; Preg Cat X

ESTRADIOL (ORAL)
(es-tra-<u>dye</u>-ole)

(Estrace)

• •

ESTRADIOL CYPIONATE, ESTRADIOL VALERATE
(es-tra-<u>dye</u>-ole)

(Depogen, Estragyn, Delestrogen, Valergen)

Side Effects

Nausea

Gynecomastia

Contact lens intolerance

Testicular atrophy

Impotence

Headache

Nursing Considerations

- Treatment of symptoms of menopause, inoperable breast cancer (selected cases), prostatic cancer, atrophic vaginitis, prevention of osteoporosis
- Contact clinician if breast lumps, vaginal bleeding, edema, jaundice, dark urine, clay-colored stools, dyspnea, headache, blurred vision, abdominal pain, numbness or stiffness in legs, chest pain, tenderness with redness and swelling in extremities
- Men should contact clinician to report impotence or gynecomastia
- Contact clinician if weekly weight gain is over 5 pounds
- Can take with food or milk to decrease GI upset
- May increase risk of endometrial cancer
- May increase risk of cardiovascular events
- Rx; Preg Cat X

• •

Side Effects

Contact lens intolerance

Gynecomastia

Testicular atrophy

Impotence

Nursing Considerations

- Treatment of symptoms of menopause, inoperable breast cancer (selected cases), prostatic cancer, atrophic vaginitis, prevention of osteoporosis
- Contact clinician if breast lumps, vaginal bleeding, edema, jaundice, dark urine, clay-colored stools, dyspnea, headache, blurred vision, abdominal pain, numbness or stiffness in legs, chest pain, tenderness with redness and swelling in extremities
- Men should contact clinician to report impotence or gynecomastia
- Contact clinician if weekly weight gain is over 5 pounds
- Give IM injection deeply in large muscle mass
- May increase risk of cardiovascular events
- Rx; Preg Cat X

KAPLAN

ESTRADIOL PATCH
(es-tra-<u>dye</u>-ole)

(Alora, Climara, Estraderm, FemPatch)

• •

ESTROGENS CONJUGATED
(<u>ess</u>-troh-genz)

(Premarin)

Side Effects

Contact lens intolerance   Testicular atrophy
Gynecomastia   Impotence

Nursing Considerations

- Treatment of symptoms of menopause, inoperable breast cancer (selected cases), prostatic cancer, atrophic vaginitis, prevention of osteoporosis
- Contact clinician if breast lumps, vaginal bleeding, edema, jaundice, dark urine, clay-colored stools, dyspnea, headache, blurred vision, abdominal pain, numbness or stiffness in legs, chest pain, tenderness with redness and swelling in extremities
- Men should contact clinician to report impotence or gynecomastia
- Contact clinician if weekly weight gain is over 5 pounds
- Apply patch to trunk of body twice a week; press firmly and hold in place for 10 seconds to ensure good contact
- May increase risk of cardiovascular events
- May increase risk of endometrial cancer
- May impair GTT results
- Rx; Preg Cat X

• •

Side Effects

Nausea   Testicular atrophy
Gynecomastia   Impotence
Contact lens intolerance

Nursing Considerations

- Treatment of symptoms of menopause, inoperable breast cancer, prostatic cancer, abnormal uterine bleeding, prevention of osteoporosis
- Contact clinician if breast lumps, vaginal bleeding, edema, jaundice, dark urine, clay-colored stools, dyspnea, headache, blurred vision, abdominal pain, numbness or stiffness in legs, chest pain, tenderness with redness and swelling in extremities
- Men should contact clinician to report impotence or gynecomastia
- Contact clinician if weekly weight gain is over 5 pounds
- Give IM injection deeply in large muscle mass
- PO: can take with food or milk to decrease GI upset
- May increase risk of cardiovascular events
- May increase risk of endometrial cancer
- May increase risk of ovarian cancer
- Rx; Preg Cat X

CLOMIPHENE CITRATE
(<u>klo</u>-meh-feen <u>sye</u>-trate)

(Clomid, Serophene)

. . . .

MEDROXYPROGESTERONE ACETATE
(me-drox-ee-proe-<u>jess</u>-te-rone)

(Provera, Depo-Provera)

Side Effects

Vasomotor flushes
Breast discomfort
Heavy menses
Mental depression
Headache
Nausea, vomiting
Increased appetite, weight gain

Constipation, bloating
Spontaneous abortion
Multiple ovulations
Enlarged ovaries with multiple
    follicular cysts
Ophthalmic "floaters," diplopia

Nursing Considerations

- Teach patient to report abnormal bleeding immediately
- Monitor for visual disturbances
- Teach patient to report pelvic pain immediately
- Teach patient to report menopause-like symptoms immediately
- Teach patient to report weight gain or edema or decreased
  urination immediately
- Patient should stop medication if pregnancy is suspected
- Rx; Preg Cat X

• •

Side Effects

Nausea
Contact lens intolerance
Testicular atrophy

Impotence
GI upset
Galactorrhea

Nursing Considerations

- Management of abnormal uterine bleeding, secondary amenorrhea,
  endometrial cancer, renal cancer, contraceptive, prevent endometrial
  changes associated with estrogen replacement therapy
- Counsel patient this medication does not protect against STDs or HIV
- Contact clinician if weekly weight gain is over 5 pounds
- Give IM injection deeply in large muscle mass, rotate sites, injection
  may be painful
- Use with caution with history of depression
- Contact clinician if swelling in calves, sudden chest pain, or SOB
- May increase risk of cardiovascular events
- May increase risk of ovarian and breast cancer
- May impair glucose metabolism; monitor blood sugars in diabetic
  patients
- Rx; Preg Cat X

The Joint Commission on Accreditation of Healthcare List of "Do Not Use" Abbreviations

One hundred percent compliance, in all forms of clinical documentation, with a reasonably comprehensive list of prohibited "dangerous" abbreviations, acronyms, and symbols continues to be the long-term objective of the Joint Commission. The following items must be included on each accredited organization's "do not use" list as of May 2005:

Abbreviation	Potential Problem	Preferred Term
U (for unit)	Mistaken for "0" (zero), the number "4" (four), or "cc"	Write "unit"
IU (for International Unit)	Mistaken for "IV" (intravenous) or the number "10" (ten)	Write "International Unit"
Q.D., QD, q.d., qd (daily) Q.O.D., QOD, q.o.d., qod (every other day)	Mistaken for each other; the period after the Q can be mistaken for an "I" and the "O" can be mistaken for "I"	Write "daily" and "every other day"
Trailing zero (X.0 mg), lack of leading zero (.X mg)	Decimal point is missed	Write X mg Write 0.X mg
MS MSO_4 $MgSO_4$	Confused for one another; can mean morphine sulfate or magnesium sulfate	Write "morphine sulfate" Write "magnesium sulfate"

In addition to the "minimum required list," the following items should also be considered for organizational "do not use" lists. These all may possibly be included in future "do not use" list.

Abbreviation	Potential Problem	Preferred Term
> (greater than) < (less than)	Misinterpreted as the number "7" (seven) or the letter "L"; confused for one another	Write "greater than" Write "less than"
Abbreviations for drug names	Misinterpreted due to similar abbreviations for multiple drugs	Write drug names in full
Apothecary units	Unfamiliar to many practitioners; confused with metric units	Use metric units
@	Mistaken for the number "2" (two)	Write "at"
cc	Mistaken for U (units) when poorly written	Write "ml" or "milliliters"
μg	Mistaken for mg (milligrams) resulting in one thousand-fold overdose	Write "mcg" or "micrograms"

Note: An abbreviation on the "do not use" list should not be used in any of its forms—upper- or lowercase; with or without periods.

The Institute for Safe Medication Practices (ISMP) has published a list of dangerous abbreviations relating to medication use that it recommends should be explicitly prohibited. This list is available on the ISMP website: *www.ismp.org*.

Source: The Joint Commission, *www.jcaho.org*. Reprinted with permission.

APPENDIX B:
Controlled Substance Schedules

Drugs regulated by the Controlled Substances Act of 1970 are classified:

Schedule I: High abuse potential and no accepted medical use. Examples include heroin, marijuana, and LSD.

Schedule II: High abuse potential with severe dependence liability. Examples include narcotics, amphetamines, and some barbiturates.

Schedule III: Less abuse potential than schedule II drugs and moderate dependence liability. Examples include nonbarbiturate sedatives, nonamphetamine stimulants, anabolic steroids, and limited amounts of certain narcotics.

Schedule IV: Less abuse potential than schedule III drugs and limited dependence liability. Examples include some sedatives, anxiolytics, and nonnarcotic analgesics.

Schedule V: Limited abuse potential. Examples include small amounts of narcotics, such as codeine, used as antidiarrheals or antitussives.

APPENDIX C:
Pregnancy Risk Categories

The U.S. Food and Drug Administration (FDA) has assigned the following pregnancy risk categories:

Category A: Adequate studies in pregnant women have failed to show a risk to the fetus in the first trimester (and there is not evidence of risk in later trimesters) and the possibility of fetal harm appears remote.

Category B: Animal studies have not shown a risk to the fetus, but controlled studies have not been conducted in pregnant women; or animal studies have shown an adverse effect on the fetus, but adequate studies in pregnant women have not shown a risk to the fetus.

Category C: Animal studies have shown an adverse effect on the fetus, but adequate studies have not been conducted in pregnant women. The benefits may be acceptable despite the risks.

Category D: The drug may cause a risk to the fetus, but potential benefits may be acceptable despite the risks (life-threatening situation or serious disease).

Category X: Animal or human studies show fetal abnormalities, or adverse reaction reports indicate evidence of fetal risk. The risks involved clearly outweigh potential benefits.

NA: Rating is not available.

APPENDIX D:
Common Medical Abbreviations

ABC—airway, breathing, circulation

abd.—abdomen

ABG—arterial blood gas

ABO—system of classifying blood groups

ac—before meals

ACE—angiotensin-converting enzyme

ACS—acute compartment syndrome

ACTH—adrenocorticotrophic hormone

ADH—antidiuretic hormone

ADL—activities of daily living

ad lib—freely, as desired

AFP—alpha-fetoprotein

AIDS—acquired immuno-deficiency syndrome

AKA—above-the-knee amputation

ALL—acute lymphocytic leukemia

ALS—amyotrophic lateral sclerosis

ALT—alkaline phosphatase (formerly SGPT)

AMI—antibody-mediated immunity

AML—acute myelogenous leukemia

amt.—amount

ANA—antinuclear antibody

ANS—autonomic nervous system

AP—anteroposterior

A&P—anterior and posterior

APC—atrial premature contraction

aq.—water

ARDS—adult respiratory distress syndrome

ASD—atrial septal defect

ASHD—atherosclerotic heart disease

AST—aspartate amino-transferase (formerly SGOT)

ATP—adenosine triphosphate

AV—atrioventricular

BCG—Bacille Calmette-Guerin

bid—two times a day

BKA—below-the-knee amputation

BLS—basic life support

BMR—basal metabolic rate

BP—blood pressure

BPH—benign prostatic hypertrophy

bpm—beats per minute

BPR—bathroom privileges

BSA—body surface area

BUN—blood, urea, nitrogen

C—centigrade, Celsius

c—with

Ca—calcium

CA—cancer

CABG—coronary artery bypass graft

CAD—coronary artery disease

CAPD—continuous ambulatory peritoneal dialysis

caps—capsules

CBC—complete blood count

CC—chief complaint

CCU—coronary care unit, critical care unit

CDC—Centers for Disease Control and Prevention

CHF—congestive heart failure

CK—creatine kinase

Cl—chloride

CLL—chronic lymphocytic leukemia

cm—centimeter

CMV—cytomegalovirus infection

CNS—central nervous system

CO—carbon monoxide, cardiac output

CO_2—carbon dioxide

comp—compound

cont—continuous

COPD—chronic obstructive pulmonary disease

CP—cerebral palsy

CPAP—continuous positive airway pressure

CPK—creatine phosphokinase

CPR—cardiopulmonary resuscitation

CRP—C-reactive protein

C&S—culture and sensitivity

CSF—cerebrospinal fluid

CT—computerized tomography

CTD—connective tissue disease

CTS—carpal tunnel syndrome

cu—cubic

CVA—cerebrovascular accident or costovertebral angle

CVC—central venous catheter

CVP—central venous pressure

DC—discontinue

D&C—dilation and curettage

DIC—disseminated intravascular coagulation

DIFF—differential blood count

dil.—dilute

DJD—degenerative joint disease

DKA—diabetic ketoacidosis

dL—deciliter (100 mL)

DM—diabetes mellitus

DNA—deoxyribonucleic acid

DNR—do not resuscitate

DO—doctor of osteopathy

DOE—dyspnea on exertion

DPT—vaccine for diphtheria, pertussis, tetanus

Dr.—doctor

DVT—deep vein thrombosis

D/W—dextrose in water

Dx—diagnosis
ECF—extracellular fluid
ECG or EKG—electrocardiogram
ECT—electroconvulsive therapy
ED—emergency department
EEG—electroencephalogram
EMD—electromechanical dissociation
EMG—electromyography
ENT—ear, nose, and throat
ESR—erythrocyte sedimentation rate
ESRD—end stage renal disease
ET—endotracheal tube
F—Fahrenheit
FBD—fibrocystic breast disease
FBS—fasting blood sugar
FDA—U. S. Food and Drug Administration
FFP—fresh frozen plasma
fl—fluid
4 × 4—piece of gauze 4" by 4" used for dressings
FSH—follicle-stimulating hormone
ft.—foot, feet (unit of measure)
FUO—fever of undetermined origin
g, gm—gram
GB—gallbladder
GFR—glomerular filtration rate
GH—growth hormone
GI—gastrointestinal

gr—grain
GSC—Glasgow coma scale
gtts—drops
GU—genitourinary
GYN—gynecological
h or hrs—hour or hours
(H)—hypodermically
Hb or Hgb—hemoglobin
hCG—human chorionic gonadotropin
HCO$_3$-—bicarbonate
Hct—hematocrit
HD—hemodialysis
HDL—high-density lipoproteins
Hg—mercury
Hgb—hemoglobin
HGH—human growth hormone
HHNC—hyperglycemia hyperosmolar nonketotic coma
HIV—human immunodeficiency virus
HLA—human leukocyte antigen
HR—heart rate
hr—hour
HSV—herpes simplex virus
HTN—hypertension
H$_2$O—water
Hx—history
Hz—hertz (cycles/second)
IAPB—intra-aortic balloon pump

IBS—irritable bowel syndrome

ICF—intracellular fluid

ICP—increased intracranial pressure

ICS—intercostal space

ICU—intensive care unit

IDDM—insulin-dependent diabetes mellitus

IgA—immunoglobulin A

IM—intramuscular

I & O—intake and output

IOP—intraocular pressure

IPG—impedance plethysmogram

IPPB—intermittent positive-pressure breathing

IUD—intrauterine device

IV—intravenous

IVC—intraventricular catheter

IVP—intravenous pyelogram

JRA—juvenile rheumatoid arthritis

K⁺—potassium

kcal—kilocalorie (food calorie)

kg—kilogram

KO, KVO—keep vein open

KS—Kaposi sarcoma

KUB—kidneys, ureters, bladder

L, l—liter

lab—laboratory

lb—pound

LBBB—left bundle branch block

LDH—lactate dehydrogenase

LDL—low-density lipoproteins

LE—lupus erythematosus

LH—luteinizing hormone

liq—liquid

LLQ—left lower quadrant

LOC—level of consciousness

LP—lumbar puncture

LPN, LVN—licensed practical or vocational nurse

Lt, lt—left

LTC—long-term care

LUQ—left upper quadrant

LV—left ventricle

m—minum, meter, micron

MAO—monoamine oxidase inhibitors

MAST—military antishock trousers

mcg—microgram

MCH—mean corpuscular hemoglobin

MCV—mean corpuscular volume

MD—muscular dystrophy, medical doctor

MDI—metered dose inhaler

mEq—milliequivalent

mg—milligram

Mg—magnesium

MG—myasthenia gravis

MI—myocardial infarction

mL—milliliter

mm—millimeter

MMR—vaccine for measles, mumps, and rubella

MRI—magnetic resonance imaging

MS—multiple sclerosis

N—nitrogen, normal (strength of solution)

NIDDM—non–insulin-dependent diabetes mellitus

Na⁺—sodium

NaCl—sodium chloride

NANDA—North American Nursing Diagnosis Association

NG—nasogastric

NGT—nasogastric tube

NLN—National League for Nursing

noc—at night

NPO—nothing by mouth

NS—normal saline

NSAIDs—nonsteroidal anti-inflammatory drugs

NSNA—National Student Nurses' Association

NST—nonstress test

O₂—oxygen

OB-GYN—obstetrics and gynecology

OCT—oxytocin challenge test

OOB—out of bed

OPC—outpatient clinic

OR—operating room

os—by mouth

OSHA—Occupational Safety and Health Administration

OTC—over-the-counter (drug that can be obtained without a prescription)

oz—ounce

p—with

P—pulse, pressure, phosphorus

PA chest—posterior-anterior chest x-ray

PAC—premature atrial complexes

PaCO₂—partial pressure of carbon dioxide in arterial blood

PaO₂—partial pressure of oxygen in arterial blood

PAD—peripheral artery disease

Pap—Papanicolaou smear

pc—after meals

PCA—patient-controlled analgesia

PCO₂—partial pressure of carbon dioxide

PCP—*Pneumocystis carinii* pneumonia

PD—peritoneal dialysis

PE—pulmonary embolism

PEEP—positive end-expiratory pressure

PERRLA—pupils equal, round, react to light and accommodation

PET—postural emission tomography

PFT—pulmonary function tests

pH—hydrogen ion concentration

PID—pelvic inflammatory disease

PKD—polycystic disease

PKU—phenylketonuria

PMS—premenstrual syndrome

PND—paroxysmal nocturnal dyspnea

PO, po—by mouth

PO₂—partial pressure of oxygen

PPD—positive purified protein derivative (of tuberculin)

PPN—partial parenteral nutrition

PRN, prn—as needed, whenever necessary

pro time—prothrombin time

PSA—prostate-specific antigen

psi—pounds per square inch

PSP—phenolsulfonphthalein

PT—physical therapy, prothrombin time

PTCA—percutaneous transluminal coronary angioplasty

PTH—parathyroid hormone

PTT—partial thromboplastin time

PUD—peptic ulcer disease

PVC—premature ventricular contraction

q—every

QA—quality assurance

qh—every hour

q 2 h—every 2 hours

q 4 h—every 4 hours

qid—four times a day

qs—quantity sufficient

R—rectal temperature, respirations, roentgen

RA—rheumatoid arthritis

RAI—radioactive iodine

RAIU—radioactive iodine uptake

RAS—reticular activating system

RBBB—right bundle branch block

RBC—red blood cell or count

RCA—right coronary artery

RDA—recommended dietary allowance

resp—respirations

RF—rheumatic fever, rheumatoid factor

Rh—antigen on blood cell indicated by + or −

RIND—reversible ischemic neurologic deficit

RLQ—right lower quadrant

RN—registered nurse

RNA—ribonucleic acid

R/O, r/o—rule out, to exclude

ROM—range of motion (of joint)

Rt, rt—right

RUQ—right upper quadrant

Rx—prescription

s—without

S. or Sig.—(Signa) to write on label

SA—sinoatrial node

SaO₂—systemic arterial oxygen saturation (%)

sat sol—saturated solution

SBE—subacute bacterial endocarditis

SDA—same-day admission

SDS—same-day surgery

sed rate—sedimentation rate

SGOT—serum glutamic-oxaloacetic transaminase (see AST)

SGPT—serum glutamic-pyruvic transaminase (see ALT)

SI—International System of Units

SIADH—syndrome of inappropriate antidiuretic hormone

SIDS—sudden infant death syndrome

SL—sublingual

SLE—systemic lupus erythematosus

SOB—short of breath

sol—solution

SMBG—self-monitoring blood glucose

SMR—submucous resection

sp gr—specific gravity

spec.—specimen

ss—one half

SS—soapsuds

SSKI—saturated solution of potassium iodide

stat—immediately

STI—sexually transmitted infection

subcut, SubQ—subcutaneous

sx—symptoms

Syr.—syrup

T—temperature, thoracic to be followed by the number designating specific thoracic vertebra

T&A—tonsillectomy and adenoidectomy

tabs—tablets

TB—tuberculosis

T&C—type and crossmatch

TED—antiembolitic stockings

temp—temperature

TENS—transcutaneous electrical nerve stimulation

TIA—transient ischemic attack

TIBC—total iron binding capacity

tid—three times a day

tinct, or tr.—tincture

TMJ—temporomandibular joint

t-pa, TPA—tissue plasminogen activator

TPN—total parenteral nutrition

TPR—temperature, pulse, respiration

TQM—total quality management

TSE—testicular self-examination

TSH—thyroid-stimulating hormone

tsp—teaspoon

TSS—toxic shock syndrome

TURP—transurethral prostatectomy

UA—urinalysis

ung—ointment

URI—upper respiratory tract infection

UTI—urinary tract infection

VAD—venous access device

VDRL—Venereal Disease Research Laboratory (test for syphilis)

VF, Vfib—ventricular fibrillation

VPC—ventricular premature complexes

VS, vs—vital signs

VSD—ventricular septal defect

VT—ventricular tachycardia

WBC—white blood cell or count

WHO—World Health Organization

wt—weight